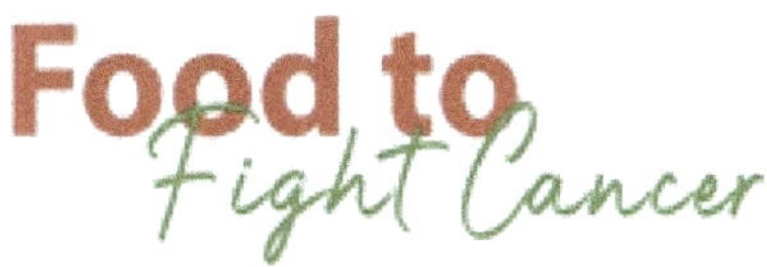

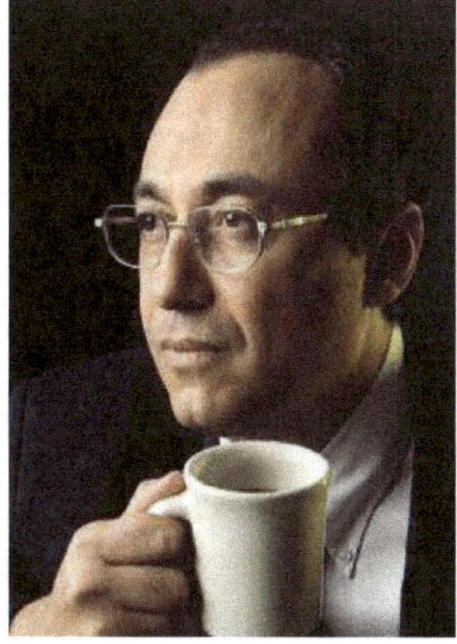

About the author:

Dr. Tarek
Abdelhamid M.D.

MLitt (Edu) is an Internal Medicine specialist and Medical Educationalist.

"Dr.Tarek" has taught medicine in several parts of the world including US, New Zealand, and the Middle East.

His lectures and ability to simplify scientific facts has been praised globally.

He developed interest in complimentary medicine after his personal experience with chronic neck pain that was relived only with natural methods.

"Dr.Tarek" believes that explaining the scientific base of complementary medicine is vital for the latter to play more role in medicine.

In this book **"Dr.Tarek"** will explain clearly how cancer develops, How food and supplements and help us in fighting this disease, and finally how to develop an effective strategy against cancer cells.

"Dr.Tarek" has developed an innovative learning model, The Multidimensional Learning Model (MDLM), to enhance the process of medical education and has been teaching conventional medicine to medical doctors and medical students for more than 30 years.

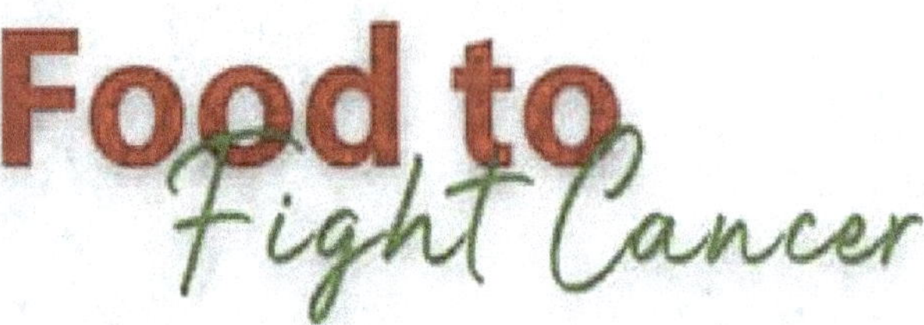

Copyright © 2023 by
Dr. Tarek Abdelhamid M.D.; MLitt (Edu)

Second edition

Dedication

The author dedicates this book to all those who currently suffer from cancer, those who suffered from it and want to prevent its recurrence, and finally to all those who want to develop a strategy to defeat it.

Dr. Tarek Abdelhamid
M.D; Mlitt (Edu)

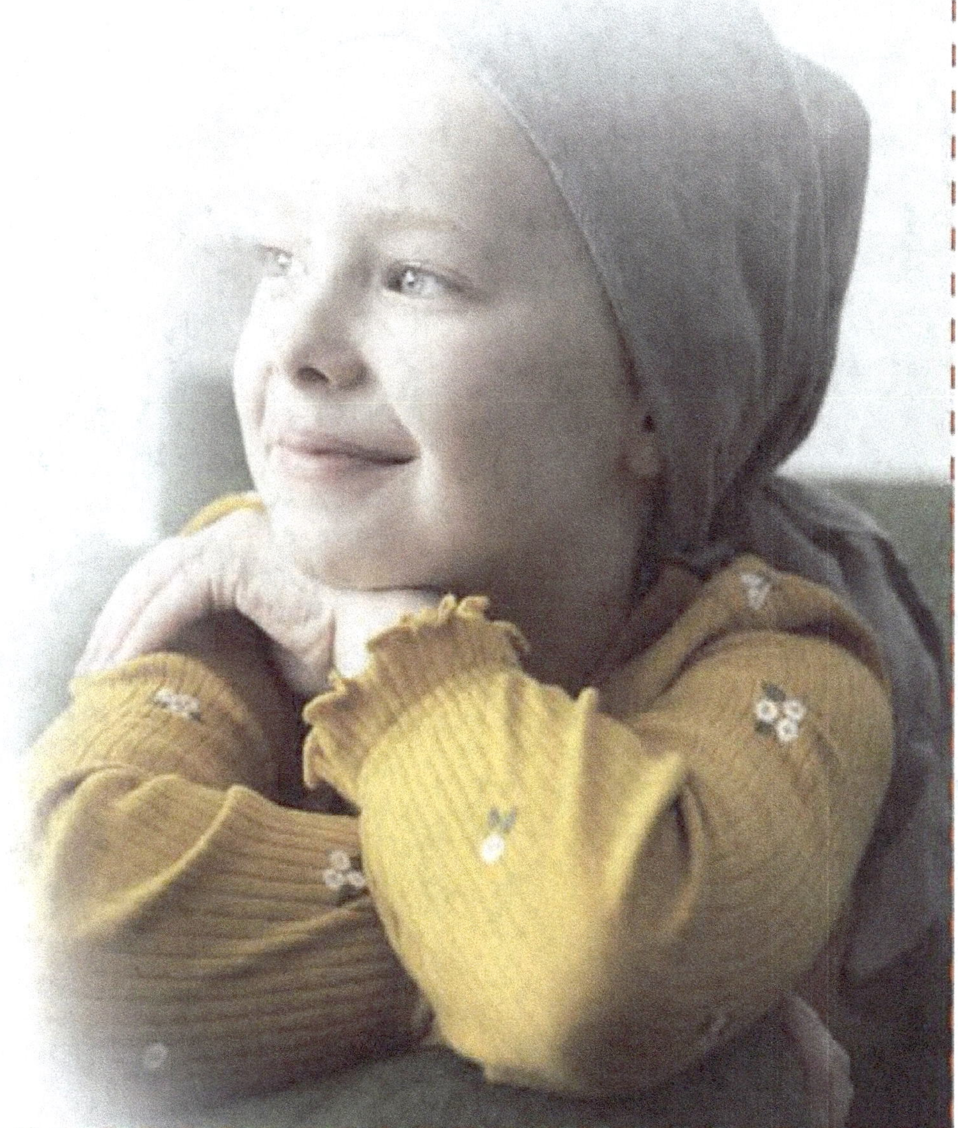

This book explains to readers how cancer develops, how food and nutrition plays a major role in fighting it and finally; how to develop an effective strategy to successfully confront this disease.

Many people ask:
Can we win
the war against
cancer

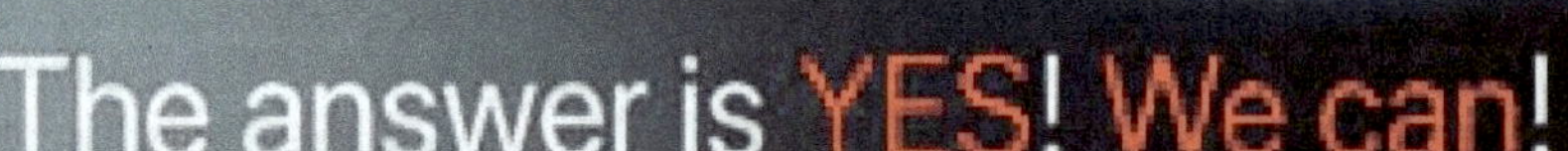

The answer is YES! We can!

Read this illustrated book to understand the role of food and nutrition in defeating cancer.

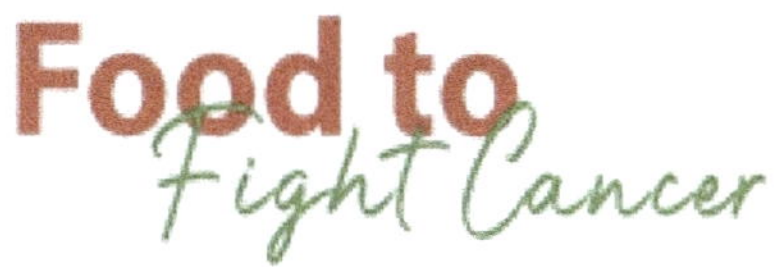

Introduction

Cancer is one of the leading causes of death in the United States. Studies into the patterns of cancer suggest that environmental factors, specifically nutrition, play a major role in its causation. There is known to be a great variation in cancer incidence based on diets.

This book discusses the mechanism of cancer formation, the role of nutritional factors in the development of cancer, and the use of nutrition and supplements as aids in fighting cancer.
It presents a complete strategy for patients on how they can use nutrition and complementary medicine in fighting cancer.

This book is designed to be a simple, fast and easy read for all those who have an interest in this topic.

Dr. Tarek uses his simple illustrations throughout to help simplify the topic for readers.

This book is for those patients who suffer or suffered from cancer and want to learn more about how complementary medical and nutritional approaches that can help them fight it.
Additionally, people who have been treated for cancer and want to safeguard against it recurring will find this book particularly beneficial for them.

Finally, this book can help all medical doctors and other health care providers understand the multidimensional nature of cancer and how nutritional factors play a major role in both the creation of this disease and the fight against it.

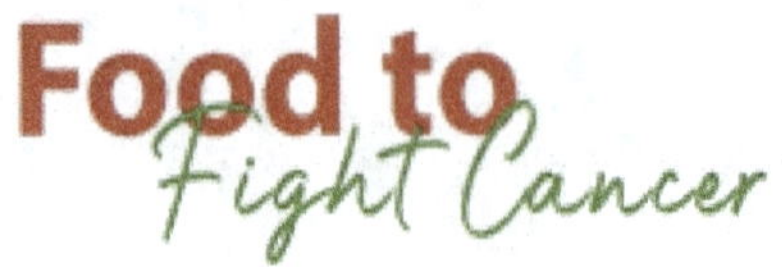

Table of contents

What is cancer?

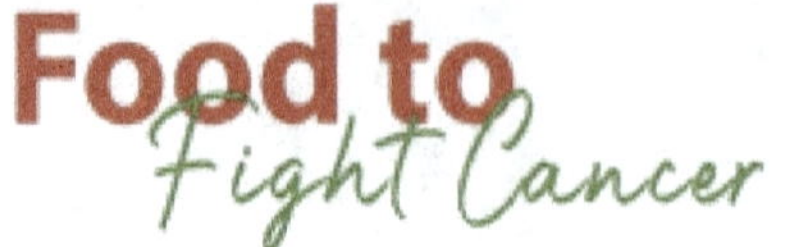

What is cancer?

Cancer is the uncontrolled division of cells in a part of the body. **Cancer** cells proliferate, invade and destroy other parts of the body, causing serious health complications.

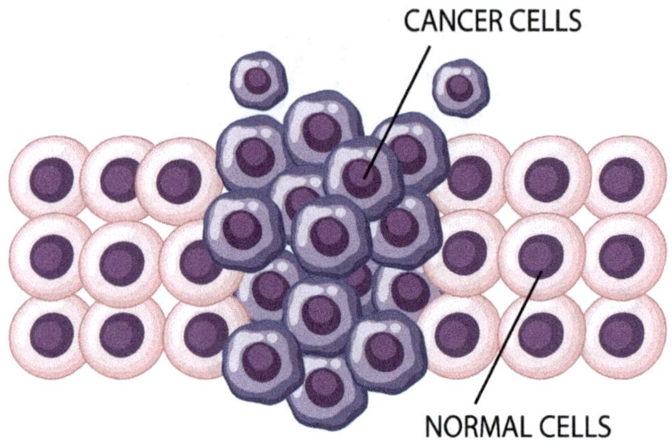

Some hormones, such as estrogen, can work as potent growth factors.
This could explain why women who use estrogen-containing pills may have a higher incidence of breast cancer, as this type of cancer depends on estrogen for its growth.

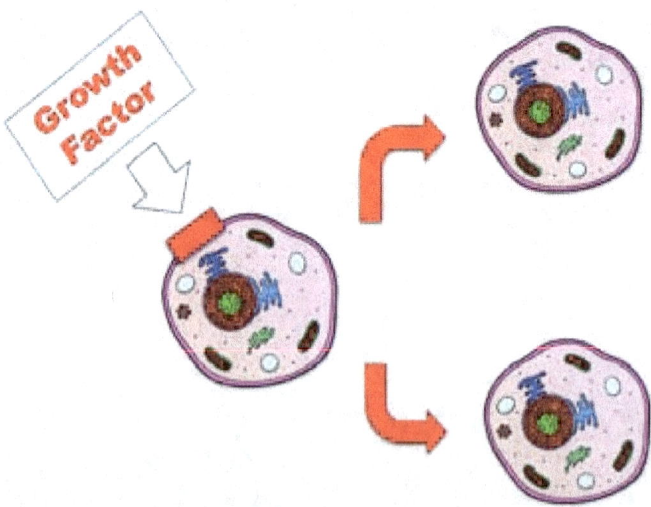

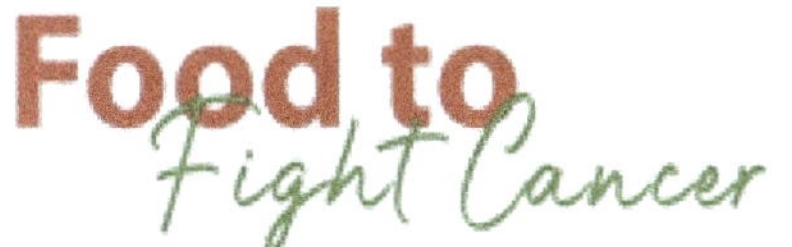

What is cancer?

At the genetic level, our DNA is activated via a specific locus called the promotor.

The promotor is controlled by an operator (regulatory gene), which is like the on-off switch for electricity.

In other words, the operator can activate the promotor (+) and increase cell division or it can inhibit it (-), decreasing cell division. Stimulation of the promotor can occur by a group of compounds called activators.

Excessive activation of our genes can lead to excessive cell division, causing **Cancer**.

Many carcinogens work as activators to our DNA whereas other biological compounds work as suppressors.

An increase in the activators or a decrease in the suppressors may lead to the development of **Cancer**.

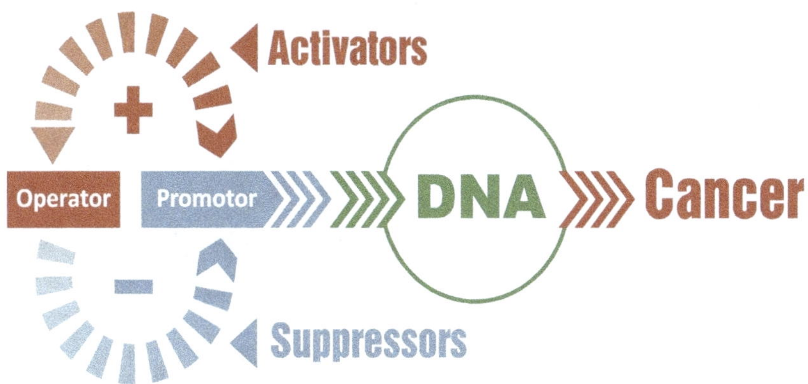

Food to *Fight Cancer*

What is cancer?

Normally, cell division is controlled by a group of genes called proto-oncogenes.

Mutation of proto-oncogenes results in the creation of oncogenes that may cause uncontrolled cell division and **Cancer**.

Many of these oncogenes work by modifying the control of our DNA at the levels of promoters and operators.

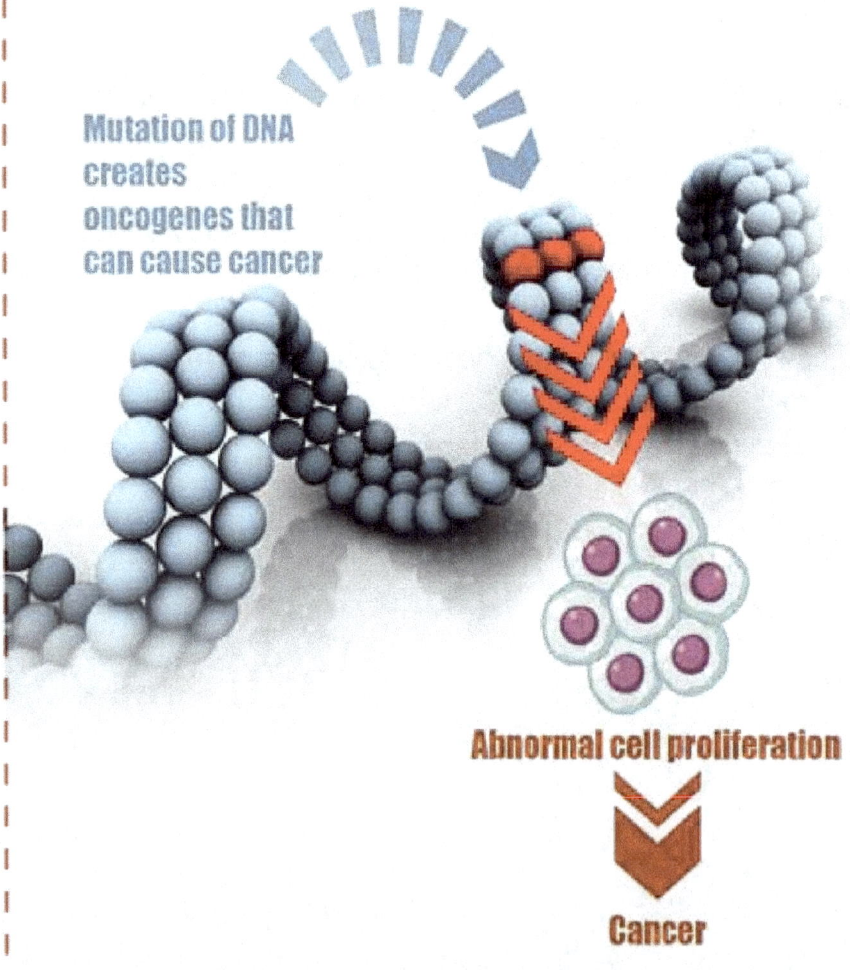

What is cancer?

Carcinogens (or external factors that may cause cancer) may cause the activation of growth promoting genes or the inhibition of the tumor suppressor genes, thus causing **Cancer**.

Avoiding carcinogens and these external factors are important in fighting **Cancer**.

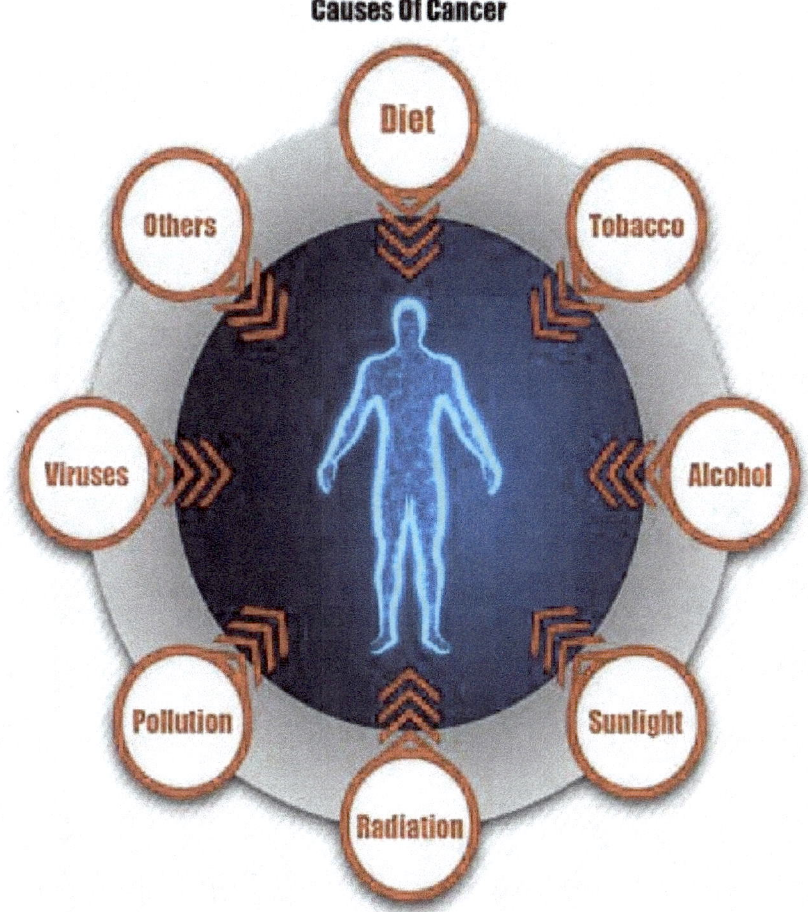

The Story of the Free Radicals

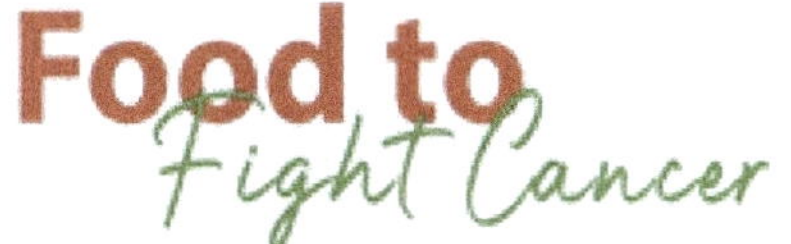

Oxidation is a reaction in which atoms lose electrons. Atoms that are devoid of electrons are called free radicals.

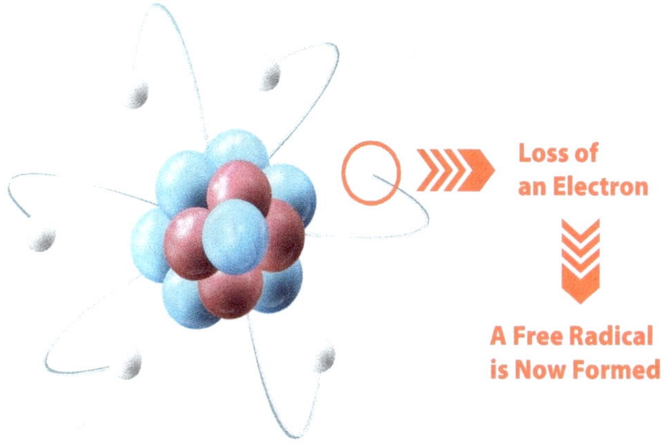

When a free radical is created in our body, it tries to steal electrons from other adjacent atoms (or molecules).
When this happens, such molecules lose their electrons and also turn into free radicals.
The process repeats itself - each free radical steals an electron from the adjacent molecule, which in turn turns into another free radical that steals an electron from the molecule that is next in line.
This goes on and on and is extremely damaging to our cells.

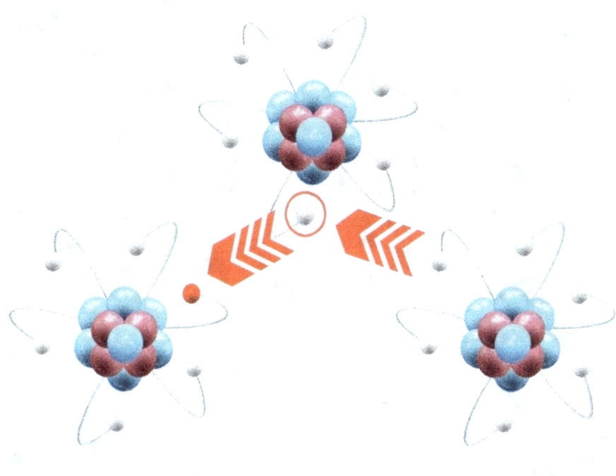

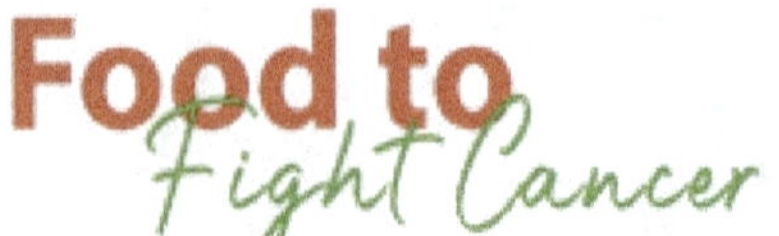

Free radicals have a special affinity with our DNA.

DNA is rich in electrons so the free radicals can easily steal the electrons that they need from it.

This causes serious damage to our DNA and thus may initiate **Cancer**.

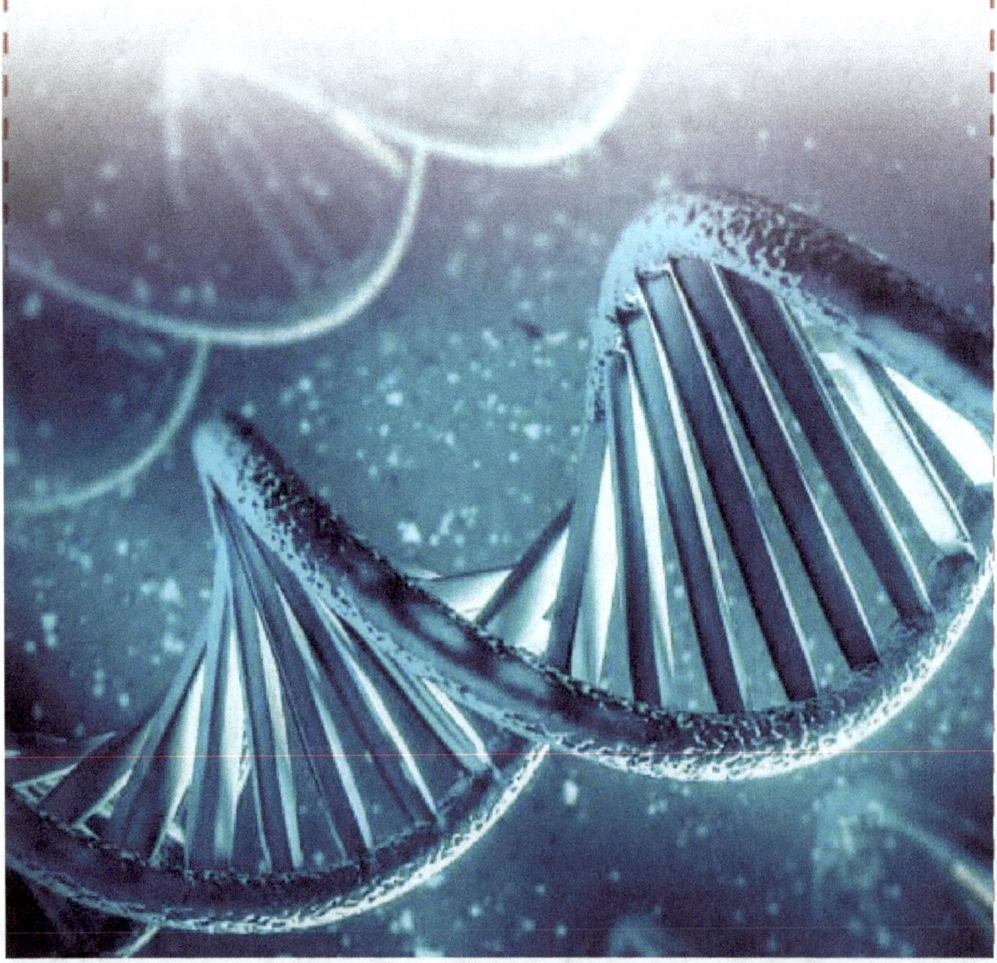

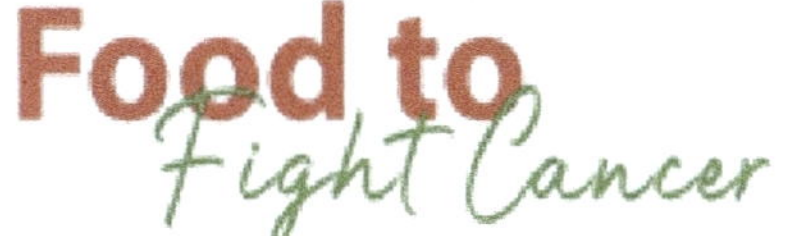

To understand the concept of free radicals, let us imagine three people - Alex, Dalia and Megan.

Imagine if all of them have an electron on their head (the apple!).

All three people in this situation are stable molecules.

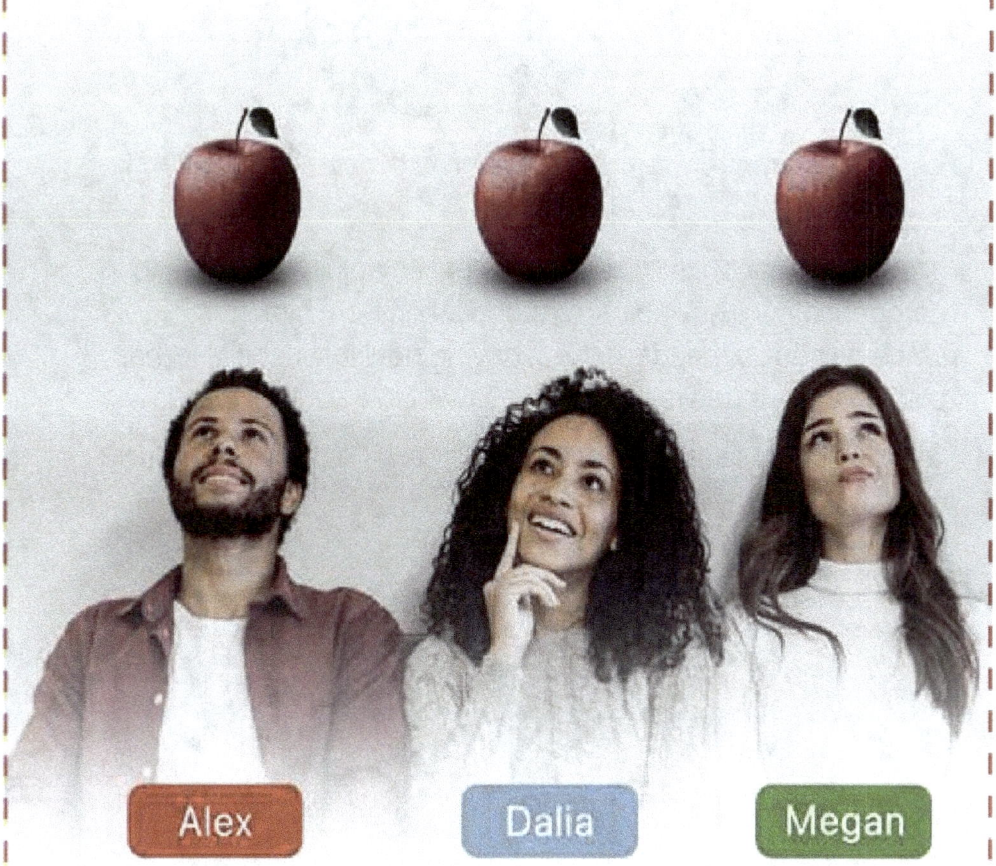

Food to Fight Cancer

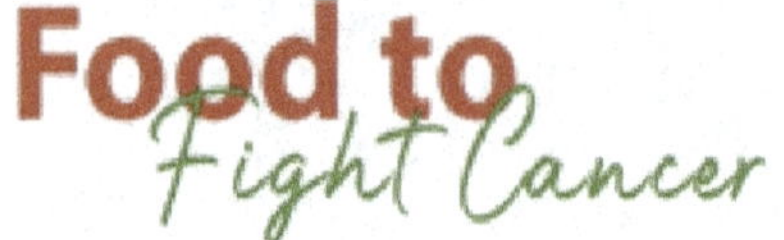

Let us imagine that an oxidative agent attacked Alex and stole his apple.
Alex finds himself without an apple and is now a free radical (a molecule devoid of electrons).

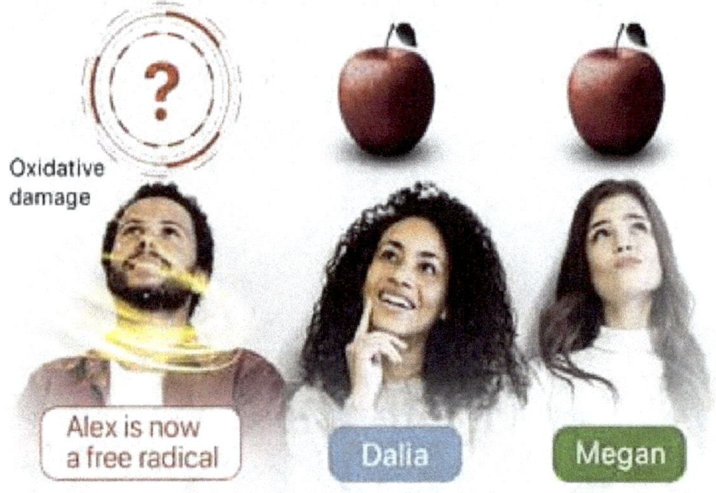

In such a situation, Alex will try to steal an apple from Dalia to compensate for having had his one taken from him.
Once he has succeeded, Dalia, having now lost her apple, has also become a free radical.

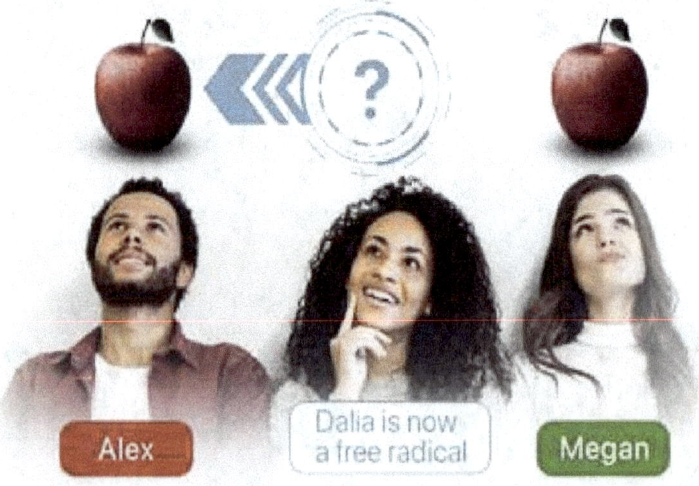

Food to Fight Cancer

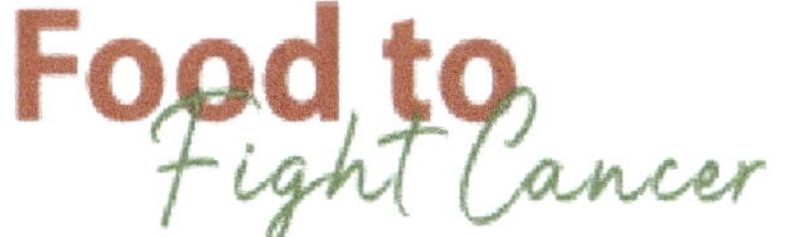

Dalia, the new free radical, will in turn steal an apple from Megan to compensate for the one taken from her.
 As a result, Megan will now turn into a free radical.

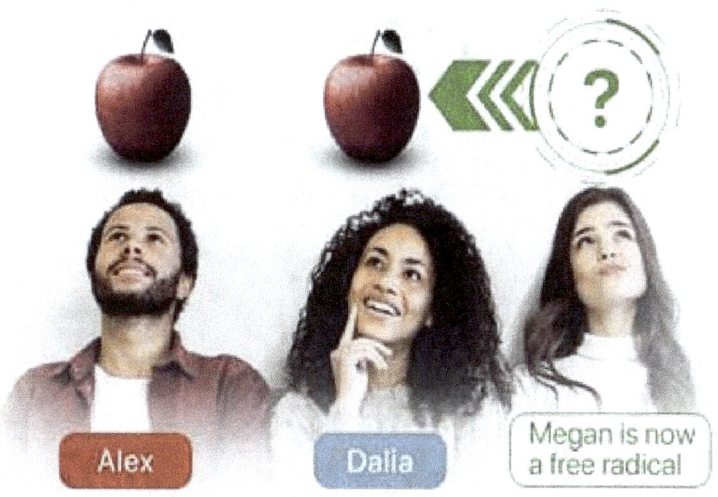

This process of each person/stable molecule having their apple/electron taken and then taking one from a person/stable molecule near them will continue until an antioxidant comes along to provide the scenario with the missing electron (giving them an apple!).

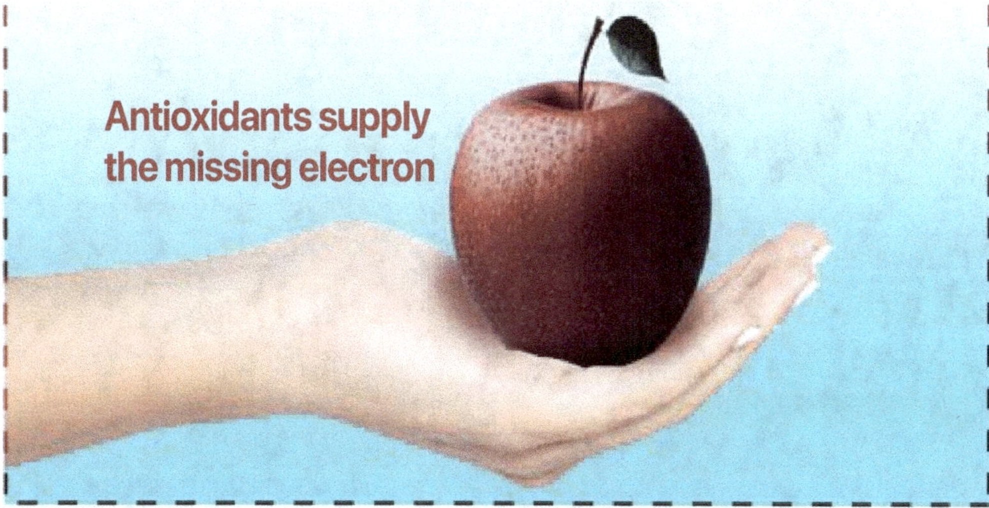

How the body protects itself from cancer

Food to Fight Cancer

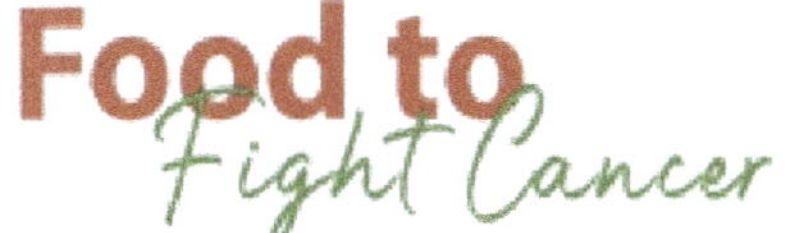

When free radicals are formed, our cells try to remove them to protect our body from their damaging effects.
Ways which can assist in the removal of the free radicals in our bodies may include the following:

1 - Powerful antioxidant vitamins, such as vitamins A, E and C
2 - Effective biological compounds, such as glutathione
3 - Enzymes that act as free radical scavengers, such as catalase (in our peroxisomes), superoxide dismutase (needs Manganese-Copper-Zinc to function), and glutathione peroxidase.

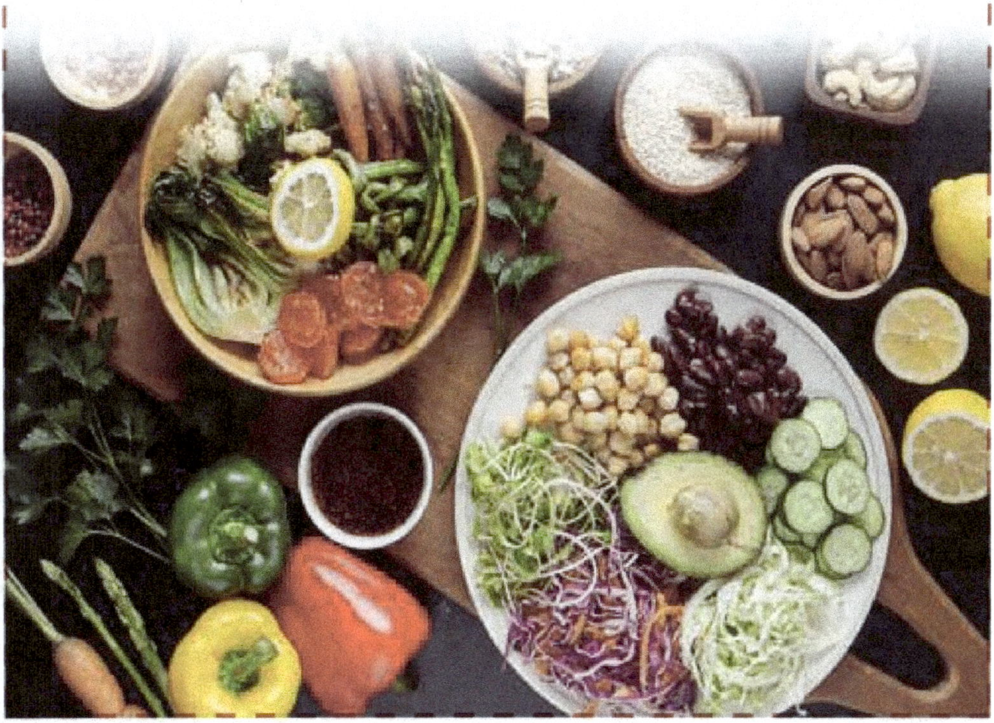

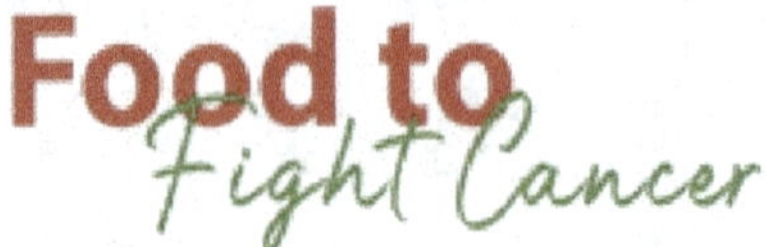

DNA methylation is a process by which methyl groups are added to DNA.

Methylation modifies the function of the DNA, typically acting to suppress gene transcription.

DNA methylation plays an essential role in maintaining cellular functions.

Changes in methylation patterns of our DNA may contribute to the development of **Cancer**.

Some bioactive food components may help fight cancer by possibly changing the DNA methylation process.

These nutrients include folate, vitamin B12, vitamin B6, methionine, and choline.

Deficiency of these dietary factors may decrease S-Adenosyl Methionine, which is a key player in the methylation process of our DNA.

DNA methylation plays an essential role in maintaining cellular functions

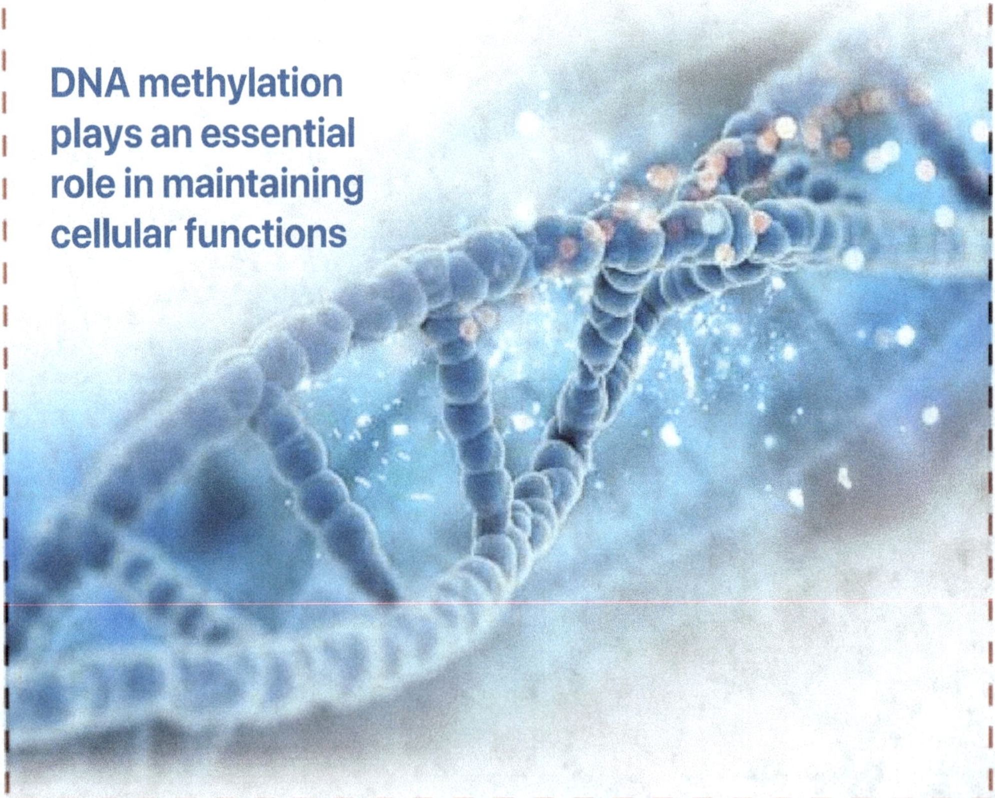

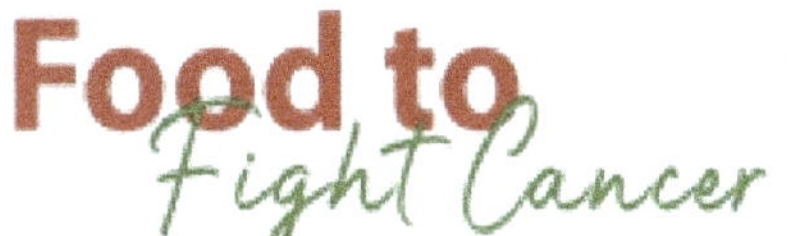

Our DNA is under constant environmental and lifestyle assaults from various directions.

The body's DNA repair genes produce many different proteins whose job is to recognize and repair damaged DNA.

Some of these proteins remove the damaged DNA while others sew up the microscopic holes caused by free radicals.

The DNA repair ability of a cell is essential to the integrity of its DNA and chromosomes.

If such repair mechanisms are impeded, our DNA can suffer from damage and unrepaired mutations, which can lead to the development of **Cancer**.

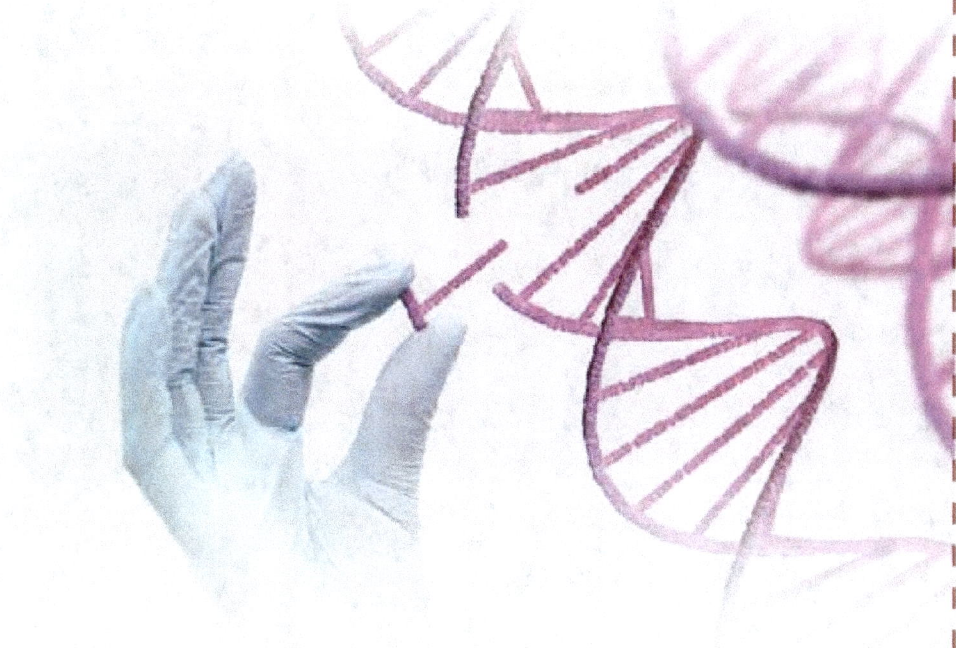

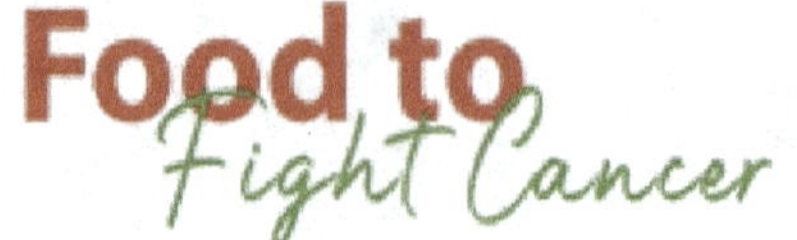

Normally, when a cell in our body turns into a cancer cell, our cellular mechanisms detect such a change and secrete an amazing protein molecule called P53.

This protein orchestrates a process called programmed cell death (or apoptosis).

Apoptosis leads to the destruction of the newly formed **Cancer** cells.

If such a mechanism is impaired, cancer develops in the body. Because of the unique mechanism of P53, it is sometimes called The Policeman of the Cell.

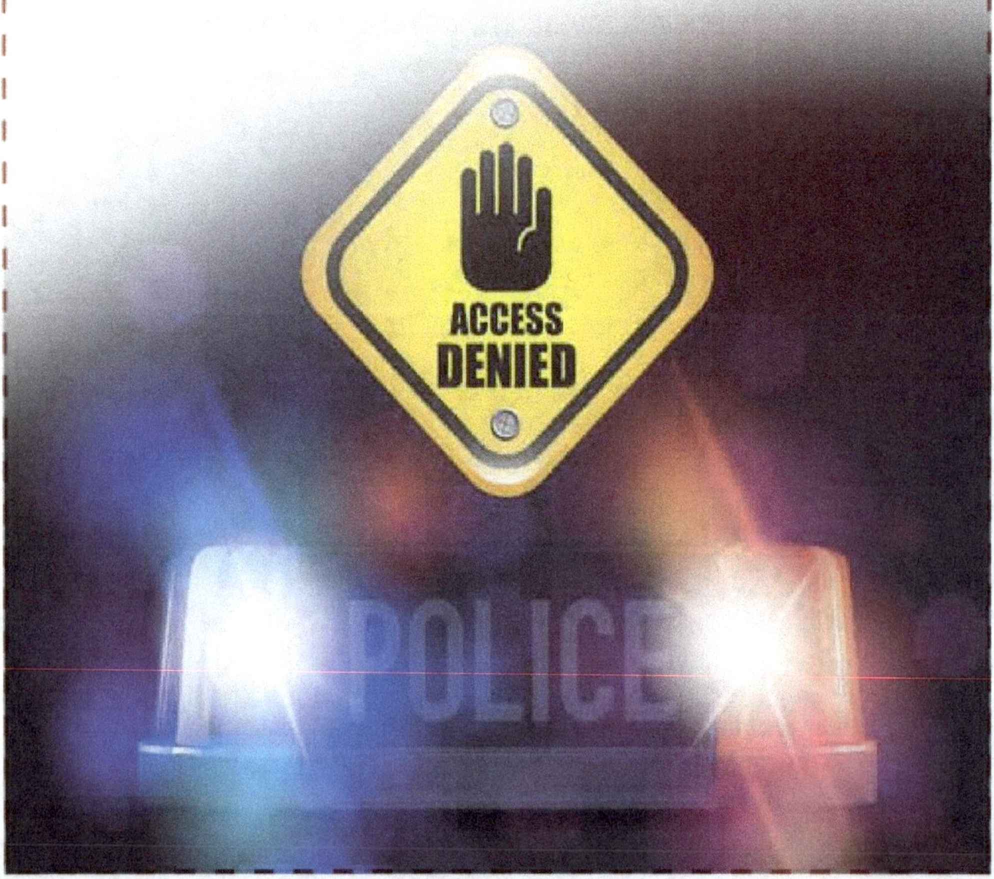

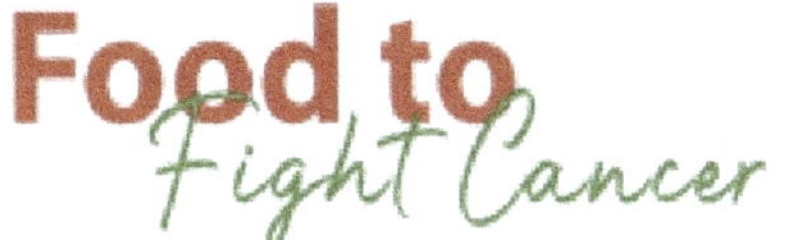

Every day, a few cancer cells develop in our body and the immune system destroys them.

If our immune system is not functioning well or its function is impaired for any reason, these cancer cells can escape and cause **Cancer**.

Enhancing the ability of our immune system can help us fight **Cancer**.

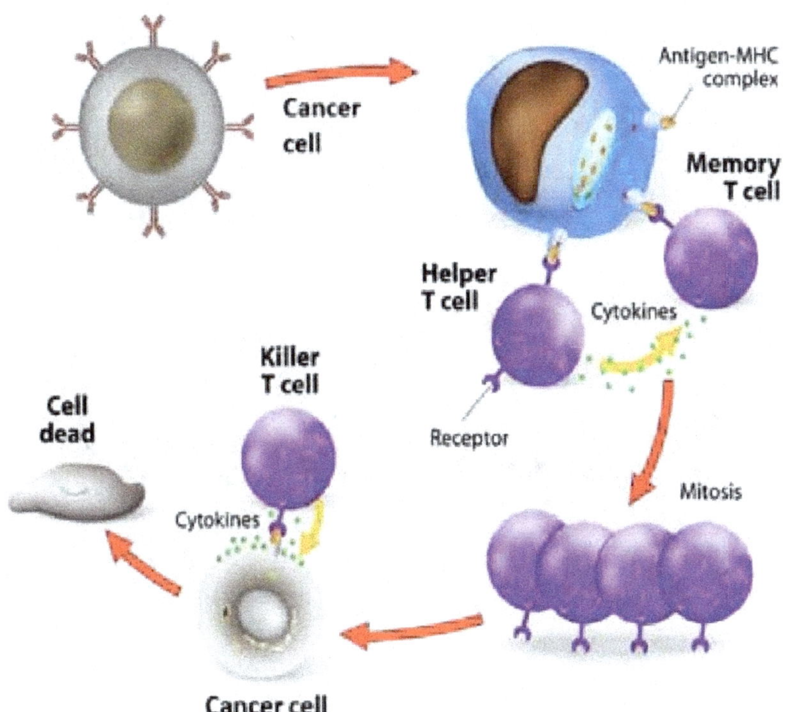

Mechanism of cancer

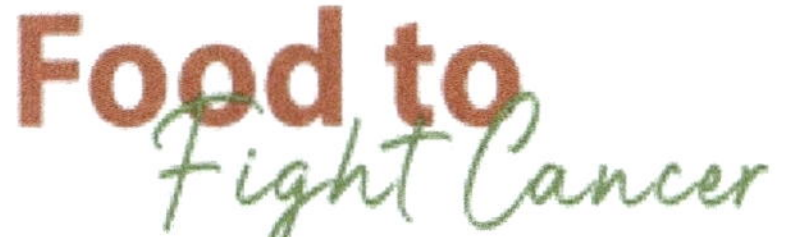

Cancer cells release certain enzymes, such as proteases, which cause degradation of collagen in the surrounding protein matrix of the basement membrane.

The basement membrane works as a barrier that prevents the spread of **Cancer** cells.

Damaging the basement membrane allows **Cancer** cells to spread.

Foods that inhibit such degrading enzymes can be extremely helpful in fighting **Cancer** as they can decrease the ability of **Cancer** cells to spread out.

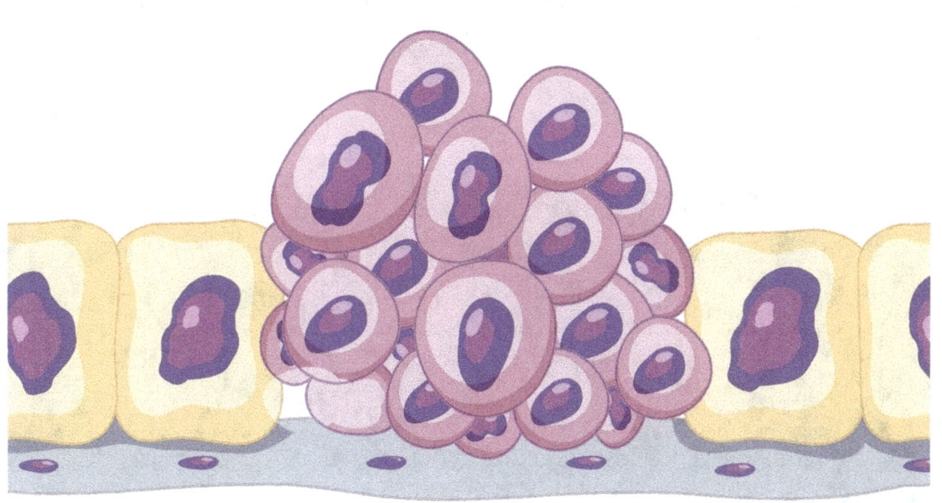

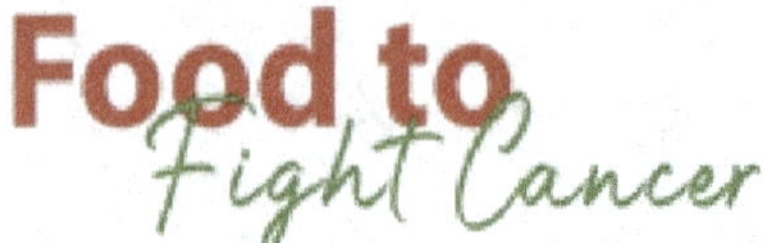

In order for cancer cells to grow and survive, they secrete certain substances to promote the formation of new blood vessels.
The formation of new blood vessels is called angiogenesis.
Angiogenesis is vital for **Cancer** cells as it allows them to receive the nutrition that they require.
As we will see later on, foods and supplements that can diminish the process of new vessel formation by suppressing angiogenesis in **Cancer** calls have the potential to be very useful agents in fighting **Cancer**.

The formation of new blood vessels is called angiogenesis

Cancer cells also learn how to evade the body's immune system so that it does not destroy them.

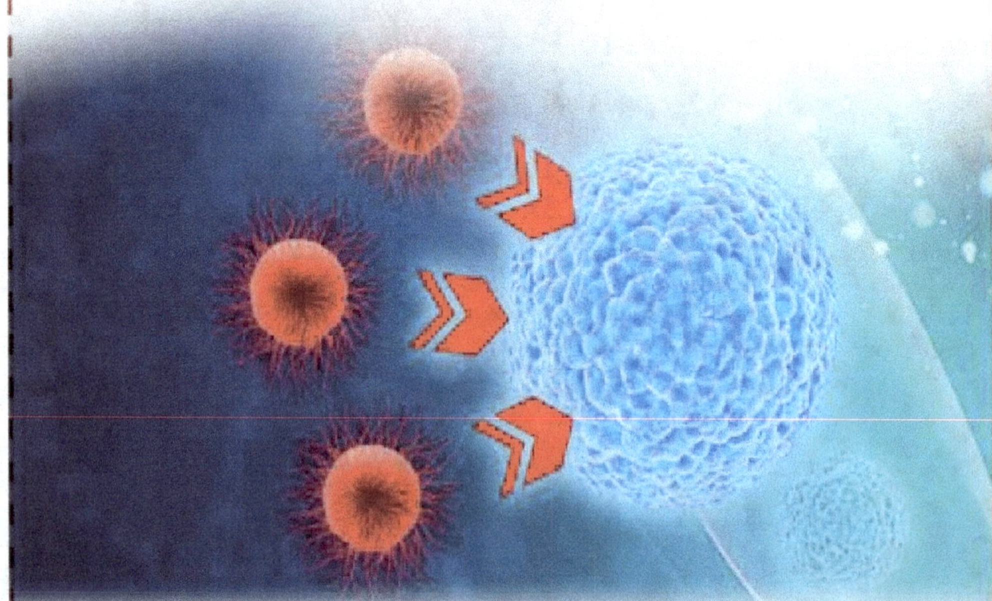

Factors that can aggravate cancer

Factors that can aggravate cancer

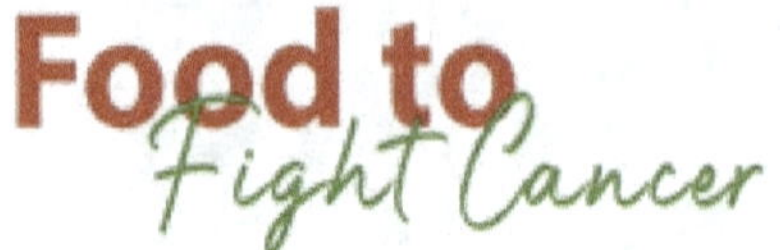

Factors that may aggravate cancer include:

- Ultraviolet Radiations (UVRs)
- Irradiation
- Industrial toxins
- Cigarette smoking
- Contraceptive pills
- Immunosuppression
- Food additives (some)
- Nutritional factors
- Viral infections
- Obesity-Stress-Depression

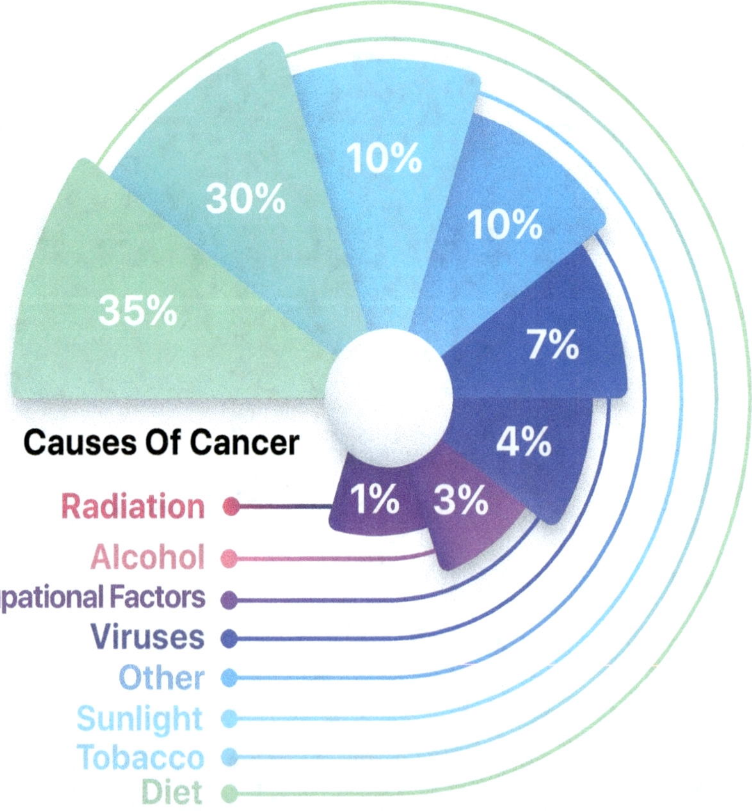

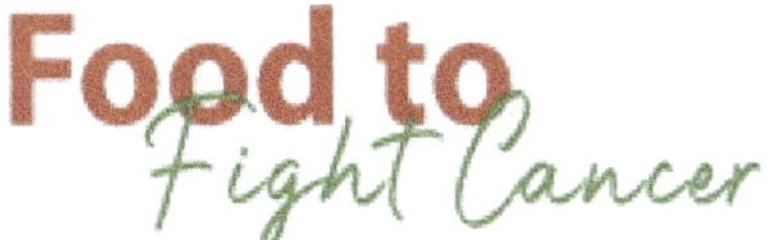

There are three main types of UVRs - A, B and C. UVB is the most damaging to our body.

The UVRs can affect our DNA bases and create what are known as pyrimidine dimers.

Such damage may cause **cancer** unless the body repairs the damaged DNA.

Excessive exposure to sunlight overwhelms our DNA repair mechanisms and ultimately may lead to **cancer** formation, especially in the skin.

VISIBLE AND INVISIBLE LIGHT

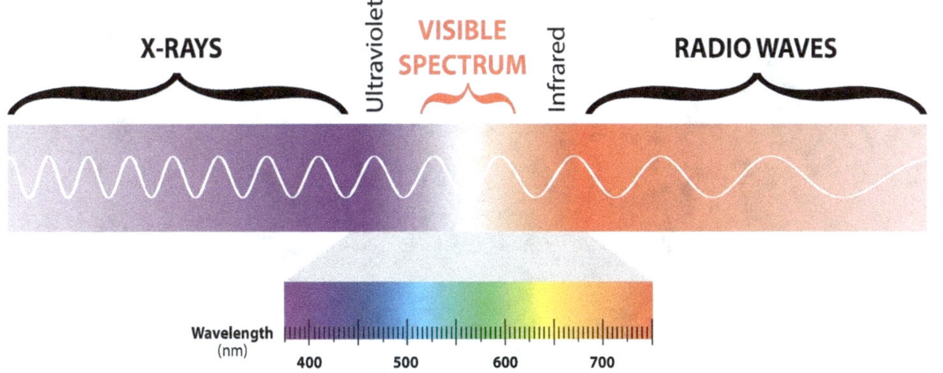

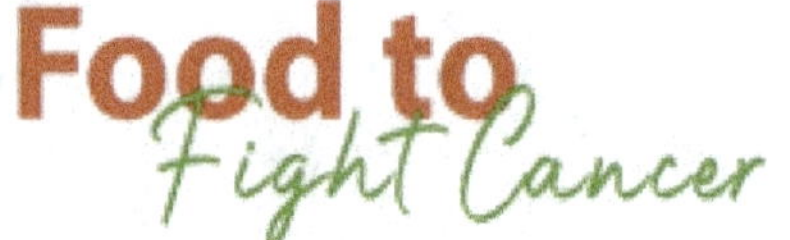

Certain infections may initiate an immune reaction against the infected cells.

If this reaction continues for long periods of time, it may lead to chronic inflammation.

The recruited inflammatory cells may release free radicals that can damage our cellular DNA and predispose to **cancer**.

The inflammatory cells may also release growth factors and other bioactive compounds that cause cellular proliferation, which may ultimately lead to **cancer**.

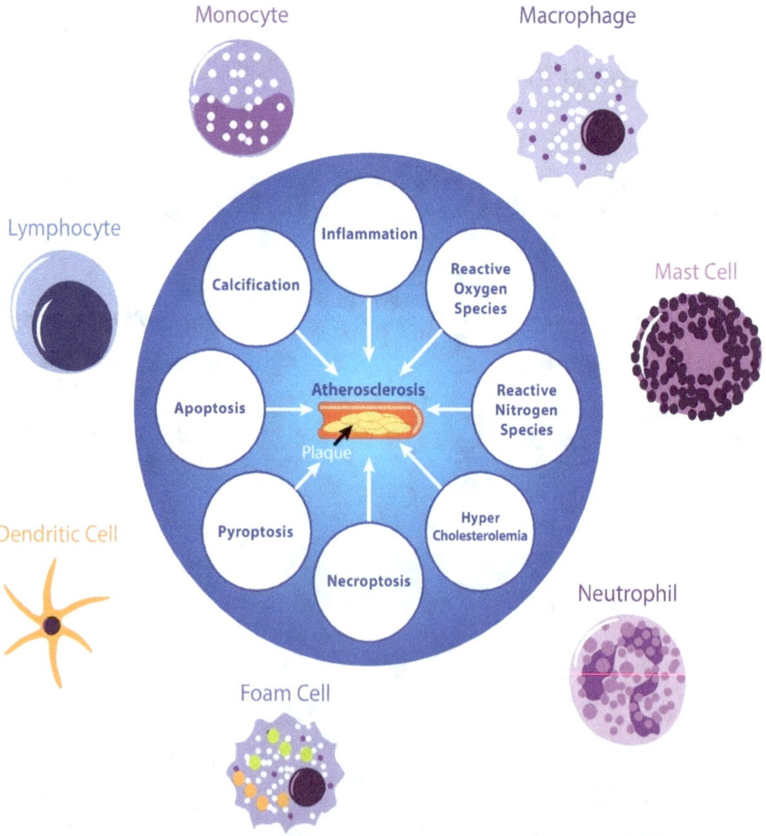

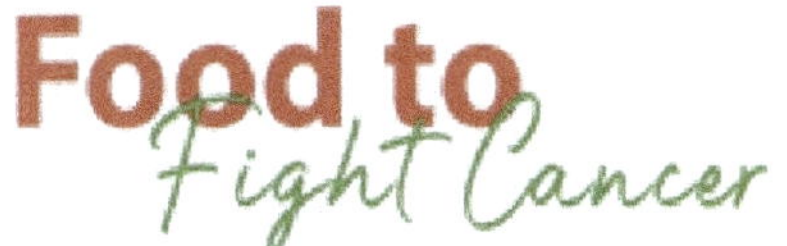

Examples of infections that may cause cancer include:
1. HBV (which causes liver **cancer**)
2. Helicobacter Pylori (which causes stomach cancer)
3. Human Papilloma Virus (HPV) (which may cause **cancer** of the cervix)
4. Epstein-Barr Virus (EBV) (which may cause lymphoma)

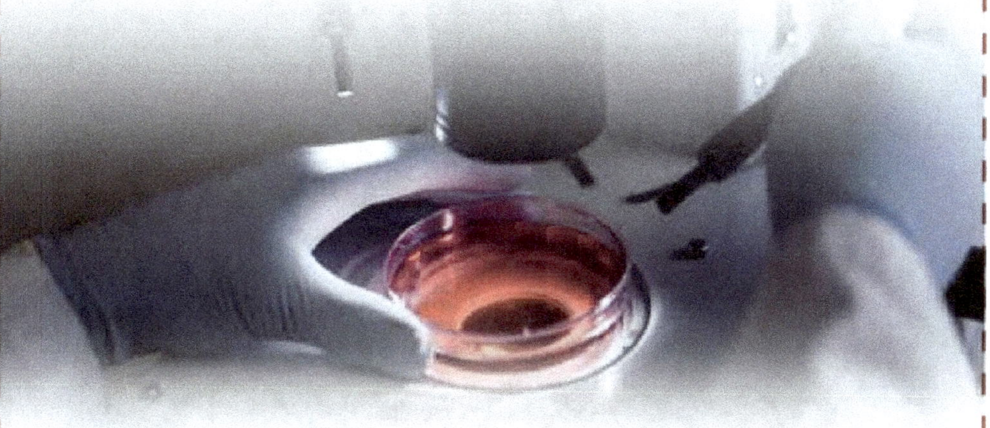

Cigarette smoking produces a substance called benzo [a] pyrene. This substance – which is formed due to the high-temperature combustion of tobacco - is highly carcinogenic.

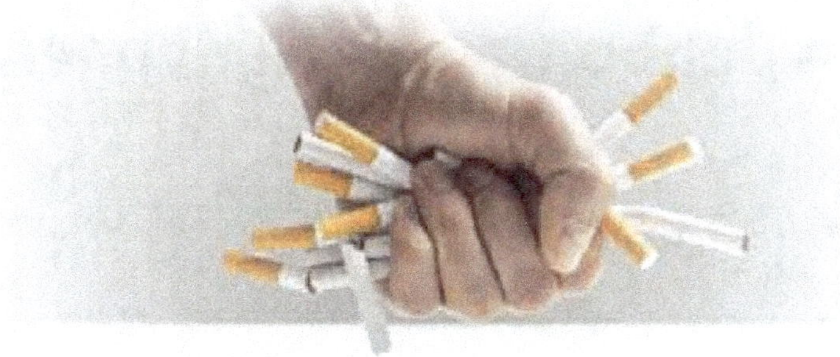

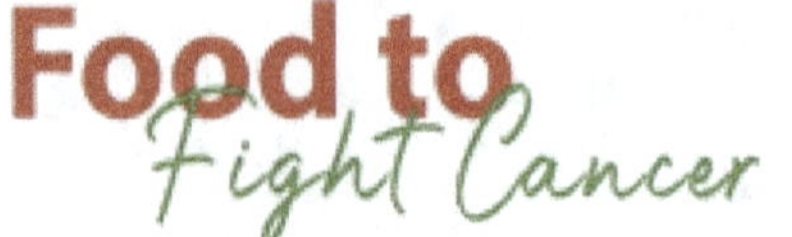

Other carcinogens (or substances that can cause **cancer**) include the hydrocarbons that are created during the process of broiling meats.

The hydrocarbons bind to DNA and initiate the process of **cancer** formation in our cells.

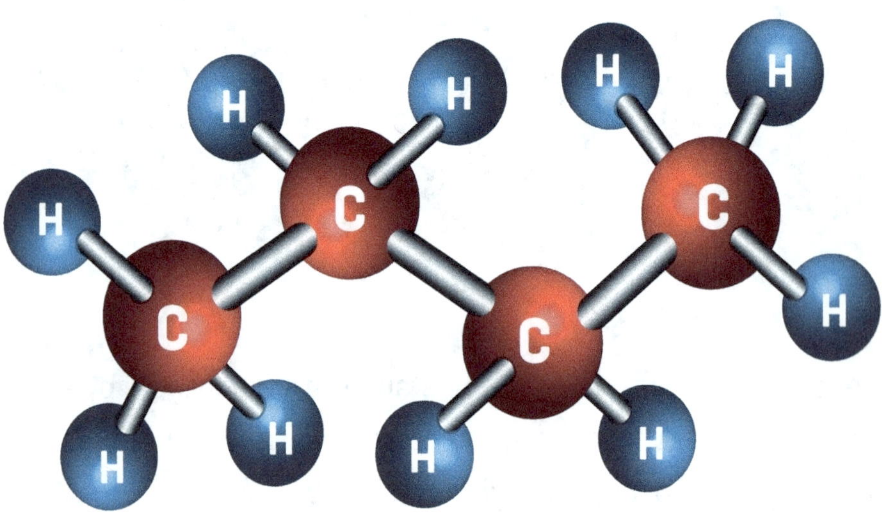

Diet
&
cancer

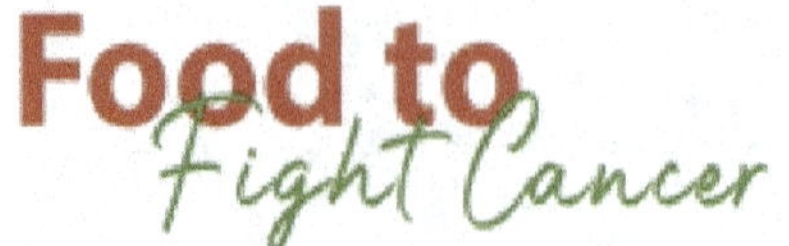

Diet may contribute to the development of cancer in several ways:

1 - Diet may contain carcinogen(s) that may affect the DNA of our cells in a way that leads to **cancer**.

2 - Some dietary components may be changed in the body to a carcinogen.

3 - Lack of dietary factors that protect us from **cancer** may predispose us to the disease

Some examples of carcinogens are aflatoxins, sodium nitrite, high animal fat intake and others.

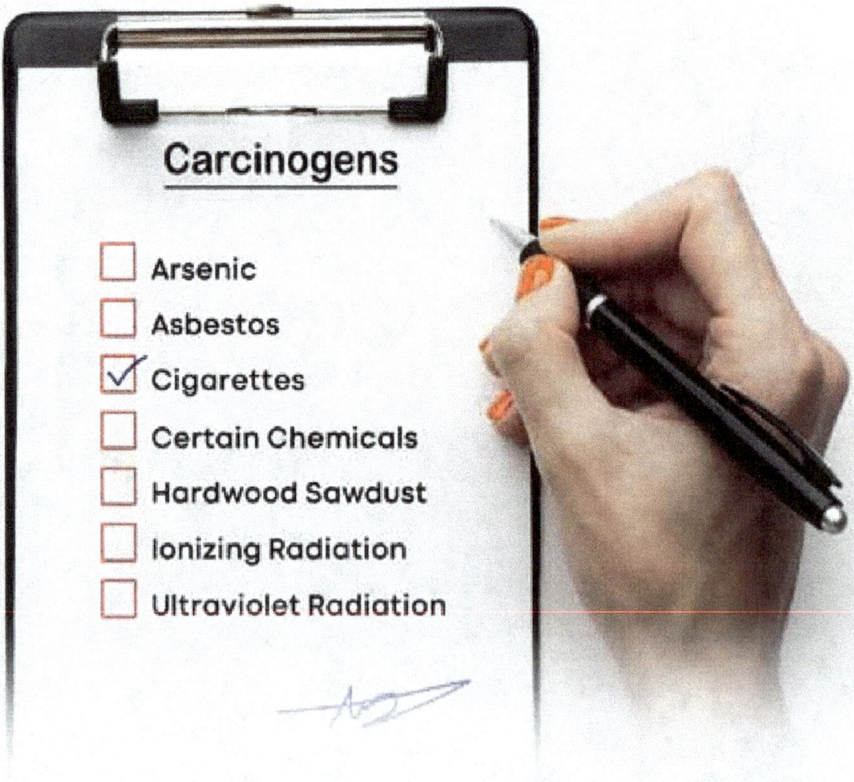

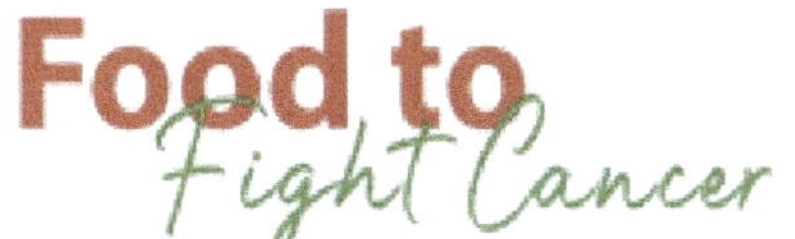

Aflatoxins are naturally occurring toxins that are produced by certain types of fungi and can contaminate a wide range of food commodities, particularly cereals, oilseeds, spices, nuts, dried fruit and dairy products.

Aflatoxins may cause specific DNA mutation that affects the production of the P53 protein in our cells.

This protects us from **cancer** as it orchestrates the programmed cell death of **cancer** cells when they are formed in our bodies.

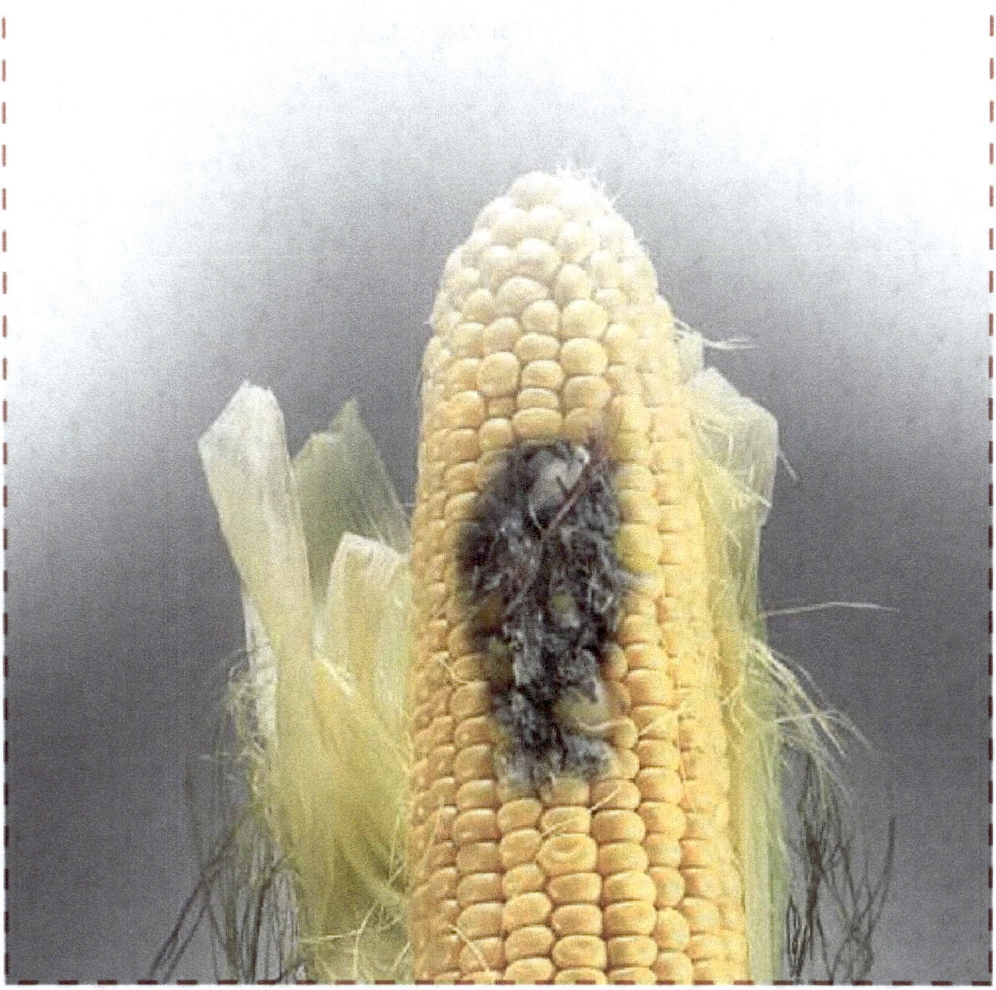

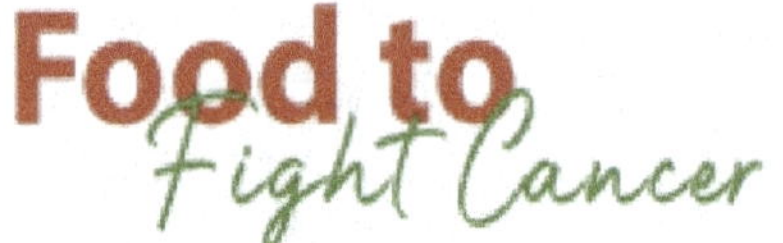

Sodium nitrite is the inorganic compound probably best known as a food additive to prevent botulism.

Nitrites are an important part in the production processes of ham, bacon and hot dogs.

The strong acidic environment in the stomach can convert nitrites in food into nitrosamines.

These have been implicated in the creation of different types of **cancer**, especially stomach **cancer**.

High temperatures, such as those reached by frying food, can also enhance the formation of nitrosamines.

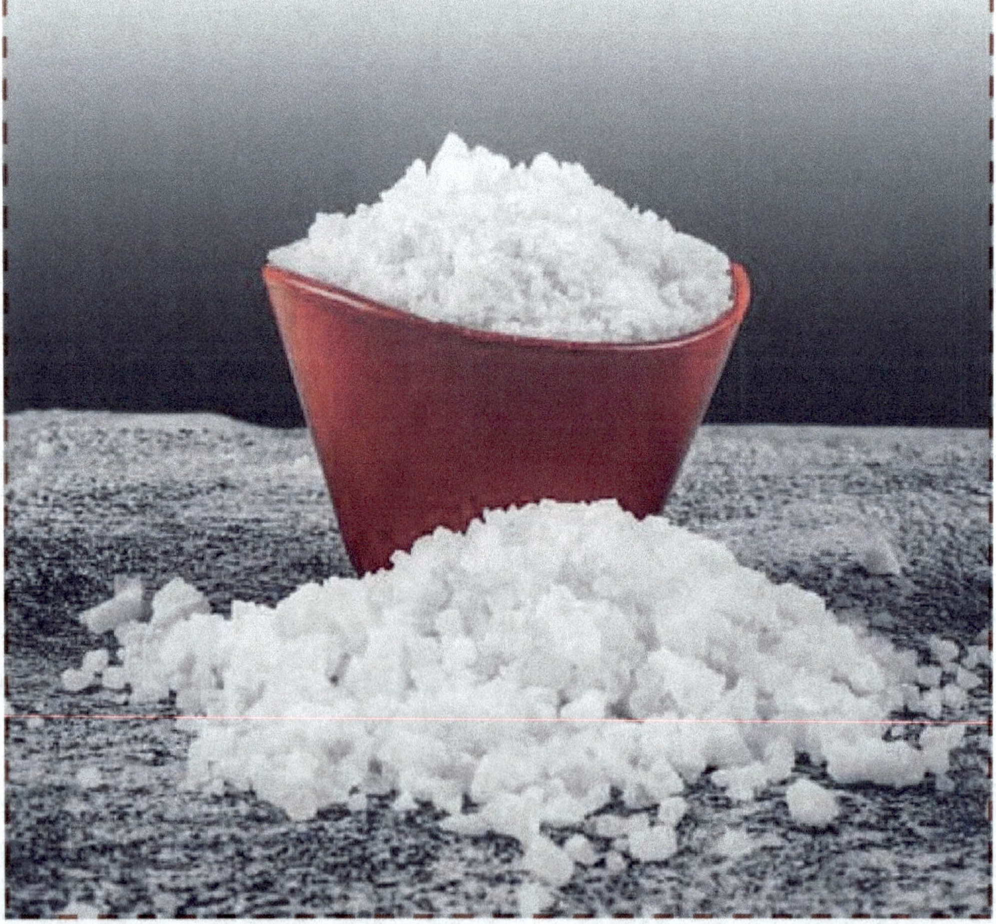

Food to Fight Cancer

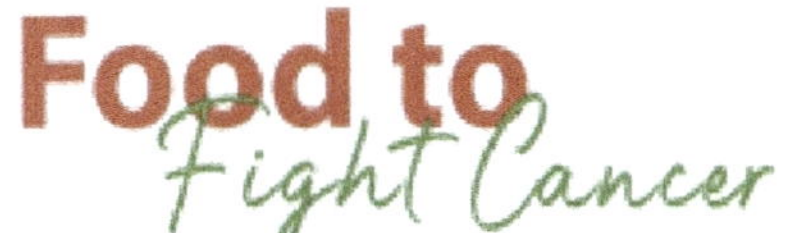

High animal fat intake may increase the body's production of bile acids, as they are needed for its absorption.

Excessive bile acid production may modify the intestinal cells (flora) in a way to favor the growth of microaerophilic bacteria.

Such bacteria may produce carcinogens in the gut, causing different forms of **cancer**.

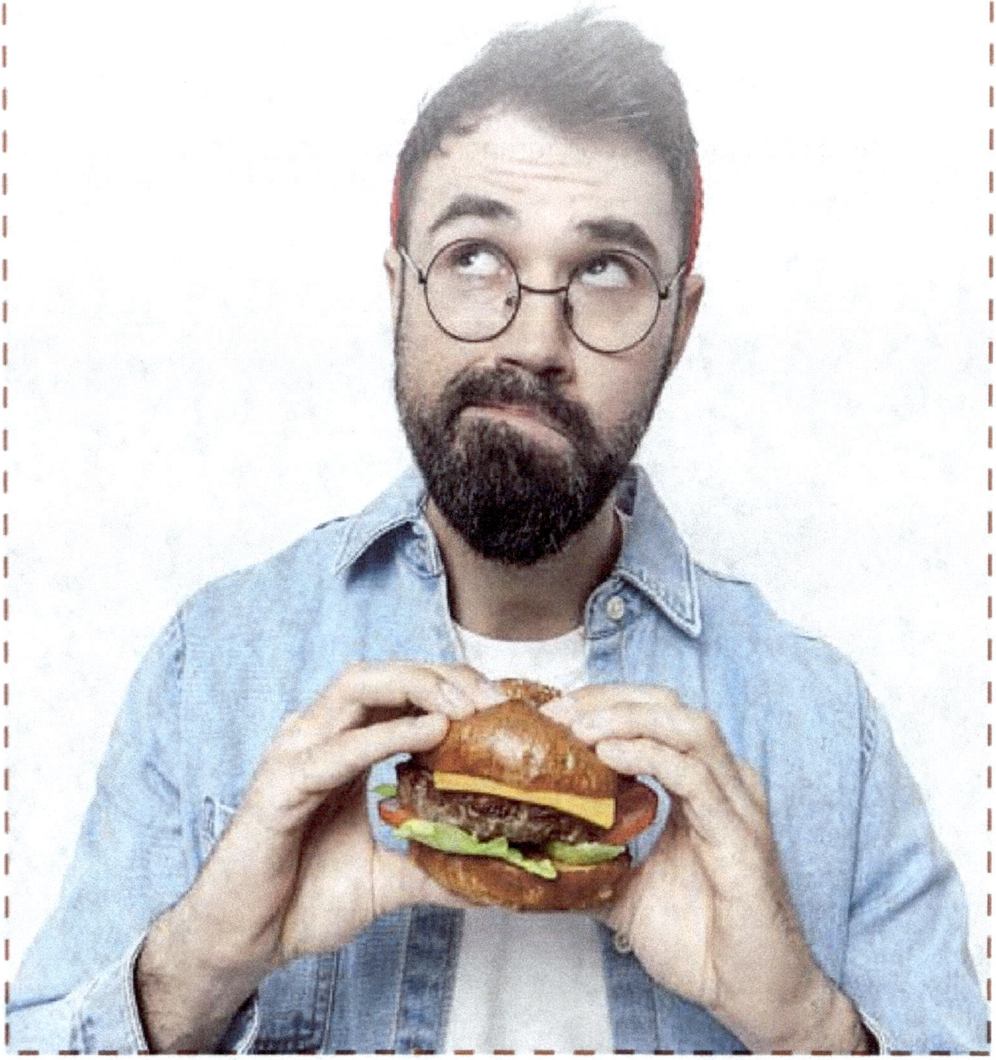

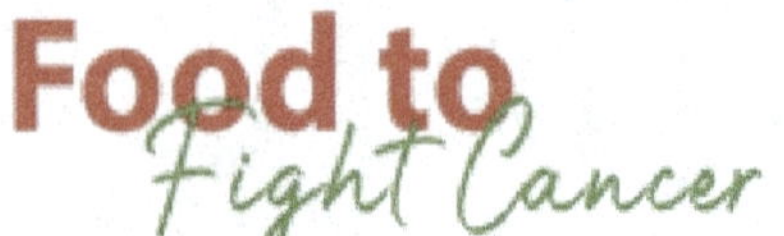

High fiber content in our diet may protect us from **cancer** in more than one way.

First: the fibers may bind some of the carcinogens produced in the gut and thus protect us from their dangerous effects.

Second: fibers may increase the stool bulk which allows the intestine to rapidly get rid of the food remnants, which may contain carcinogens.

This process decreases the time that food remains in the intestine and therefore decreases the exposure of our intestinal cells to such food remnants that contain the carcinogenic substances.

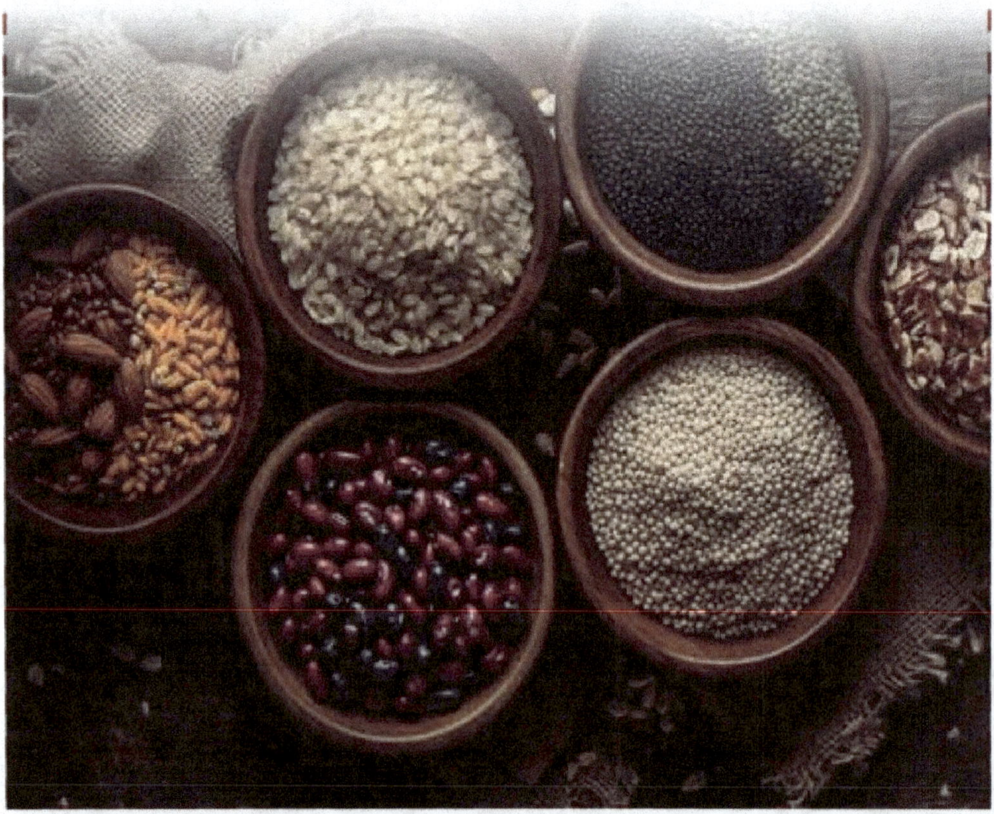

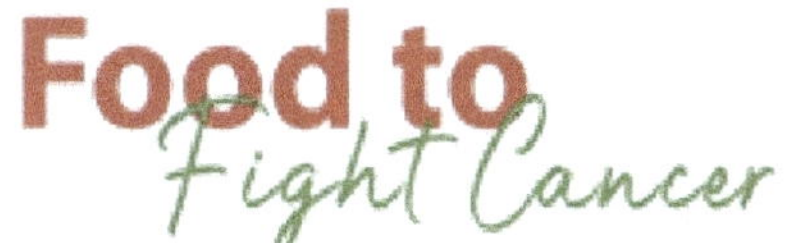

A diet that does not provide sufficient antioxidants may allow the oxidative agents or free radicals to damage our DNA molecules, causing cancer.

Antioxidants in diet include vitamins A, C and E, beta carotenes, lycopene, selenium and many other compounds.

A diet rich in antioxidants can - at least in theory - protect the body from the extremely damaging and carcinogenic effects of oxidative damage by the free radicals.

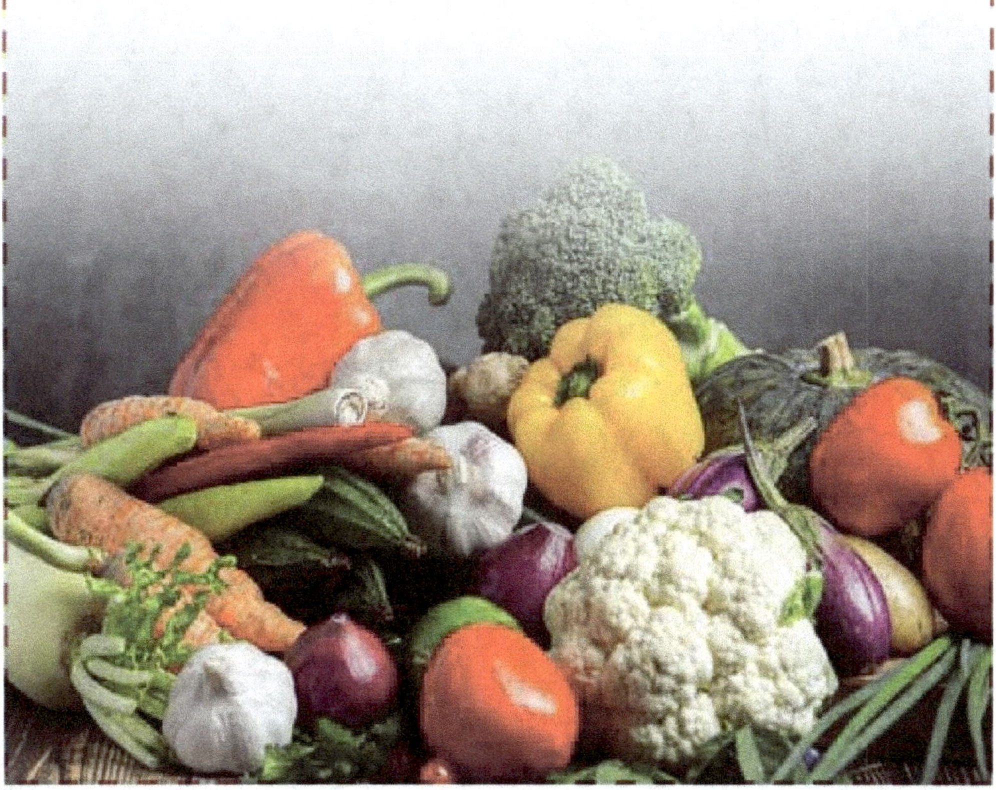

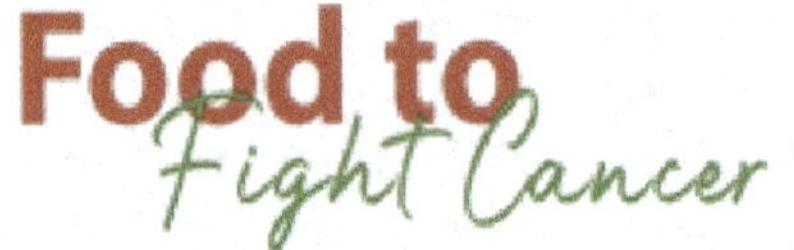

Food to Fight Cancer

Vitamin D has been found to have a number of attributes that might slow or prevent the development and progression of **cancer**. These include promoting cellular differentiation, decreasing **cancer** cell growth, activating programmed cell death of cancer cells (apoptosis), and reducing tumor blood vessel formation (angiogenesis). Vitamin D deficiency has also been implicated in the development of several forms of **cancer**.

Vitamin D can be created in our body through exposure to sunlight. It can also be obtained from dietary sources such as fatty fish (including salmon, tuna and mackerel) and fish liver oils.

Small amounts of vitamin D are found in beef liver, cheese and egg yolks. Some mushrooms may also provide vitamin D.

Currently, fortified foods are considered to be a major source of vitamin D in our diet.

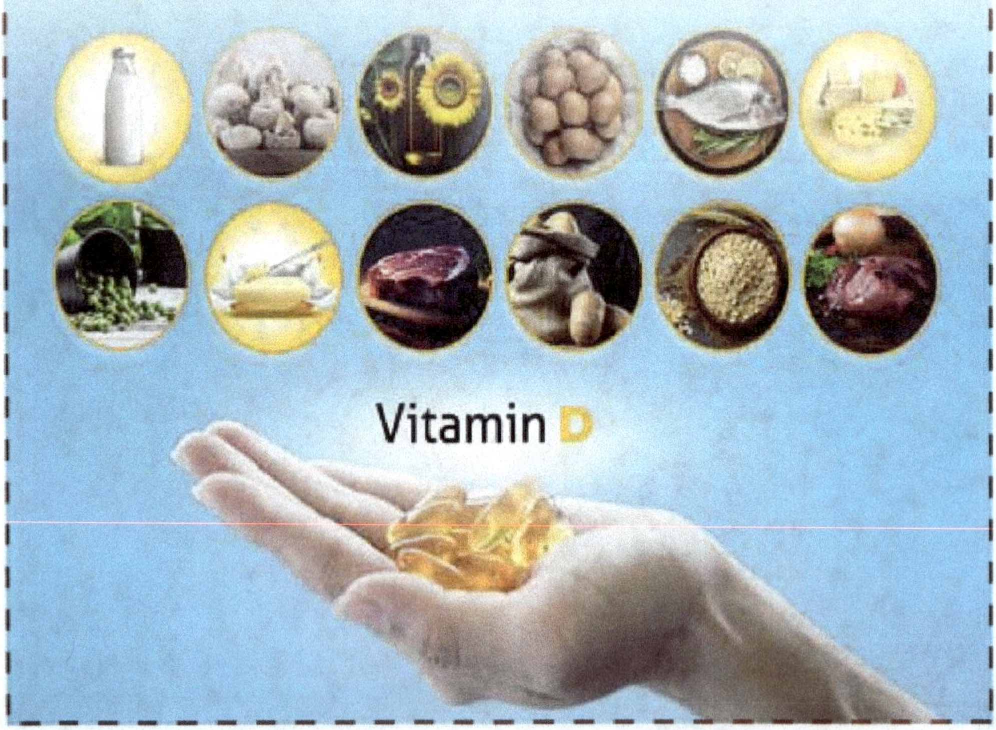

Chapter

7

Other contributing factors to cancer

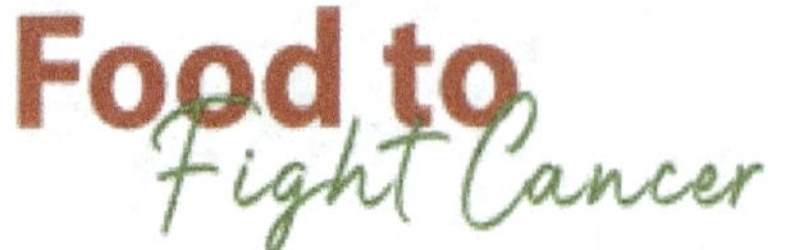

Obesity may also contribute to the formation of cancer in our body. In obesity, the fat cells are full of fat and are thus unable to respond properly to insulin.

The body recognizes this as deficiency of insulin and responds by producing more insulin (as an attempt to overcome this problem).

The high insulin levels may work as a 'growth factors' and causes activation of some metabolic pathways that can ultimately causes **cancer**.

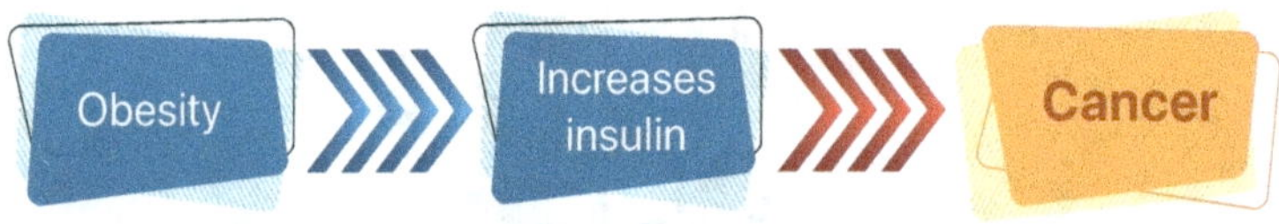

Additionally, the high insulin levels associated with obesity increases the production of a growth factor in our body called Insulin Like Growth Factor 1 (IGF-I).

This growth factor can stimulate the growth of our cells and thus result in the development of **cancer**.

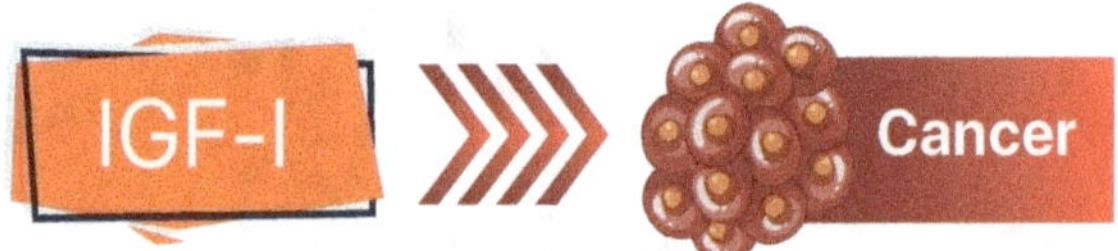

Furthermore, obesity decreases the production of Sex Hormone Binding Globulins (SHBG) and thus allows the sex hormones to circulate freely in our blood (See: the red circles in the figure below). The free sex hormones may cause excessive stimulation of our cells, which can aggravate the cancerous process.

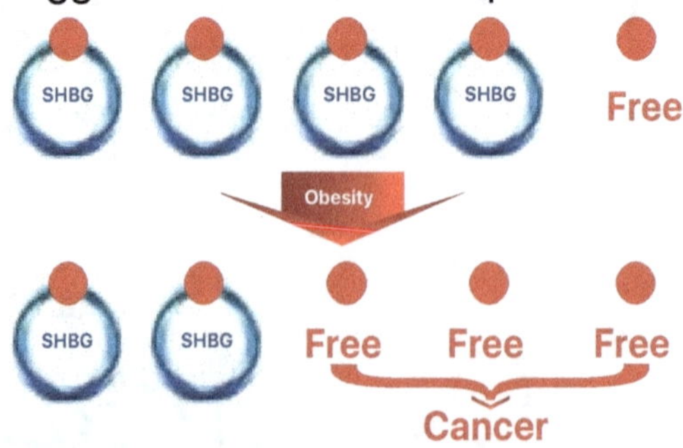

Other contributing factors to cancer

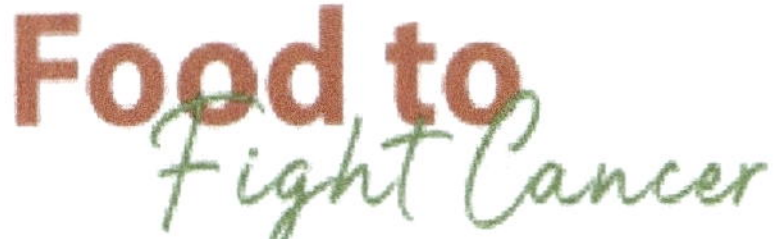

Stress can aggravate **cancer** by triggering a 'master switch' gene which allows the disease to spread.

The gene, which is called ATF3, promotes the immune cells to act erratically and give **cancer** an escape route to other areas of the body.

Additionally, chronic stress increases anti-stress hormones such as cortisone.

Cortisone can impede the function of the immune cells and thus impede the ability of our immune system to get rid of **cancer** cells.

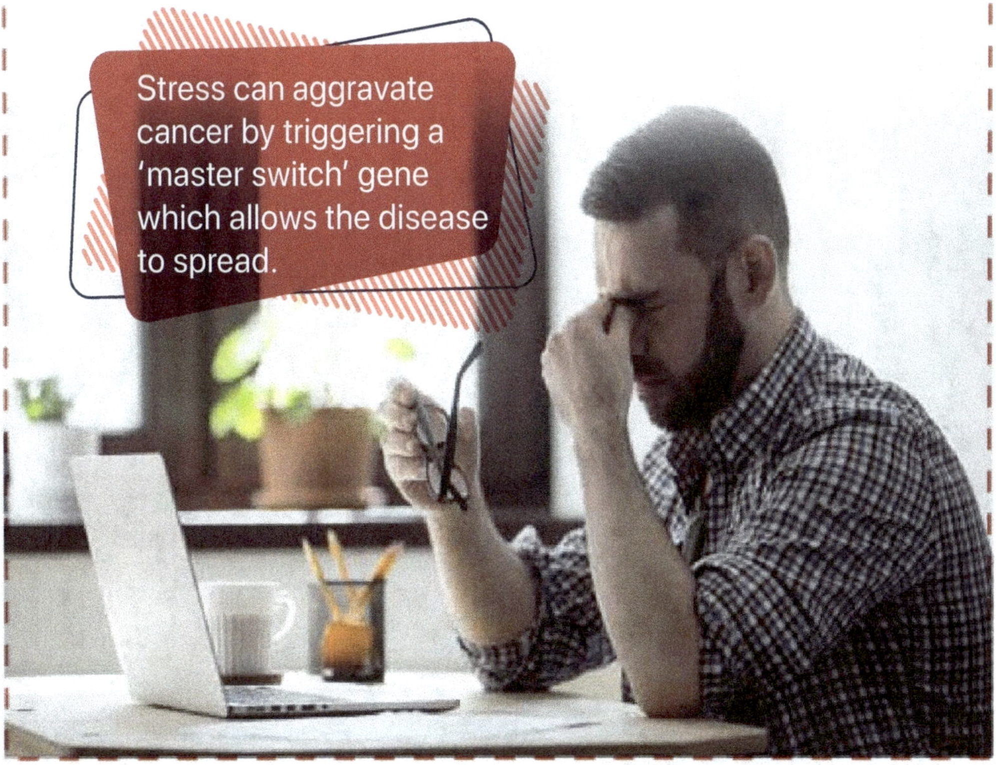

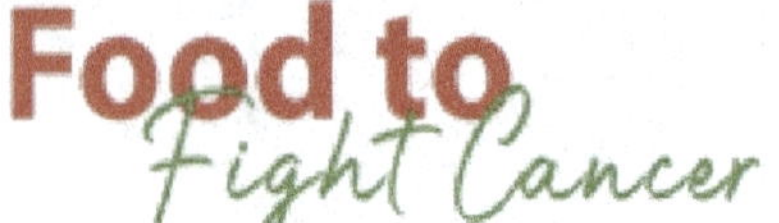

Depression has also been linked to increased cancer risk and to the shortened survival of **cancer** patients.

Depression may be associated with elevation in the concentrations of circulating plasma proinflammatory cytokines, which may mediate biological processes that aggravate **cancer**.

In addition, depression suppresses the functions of T killer cells of our immune system.

These cells naturally kill newly formed **cancer** cells in our bodies. Failure to do so effectively can result in aggravation of different forms of **cancer**.

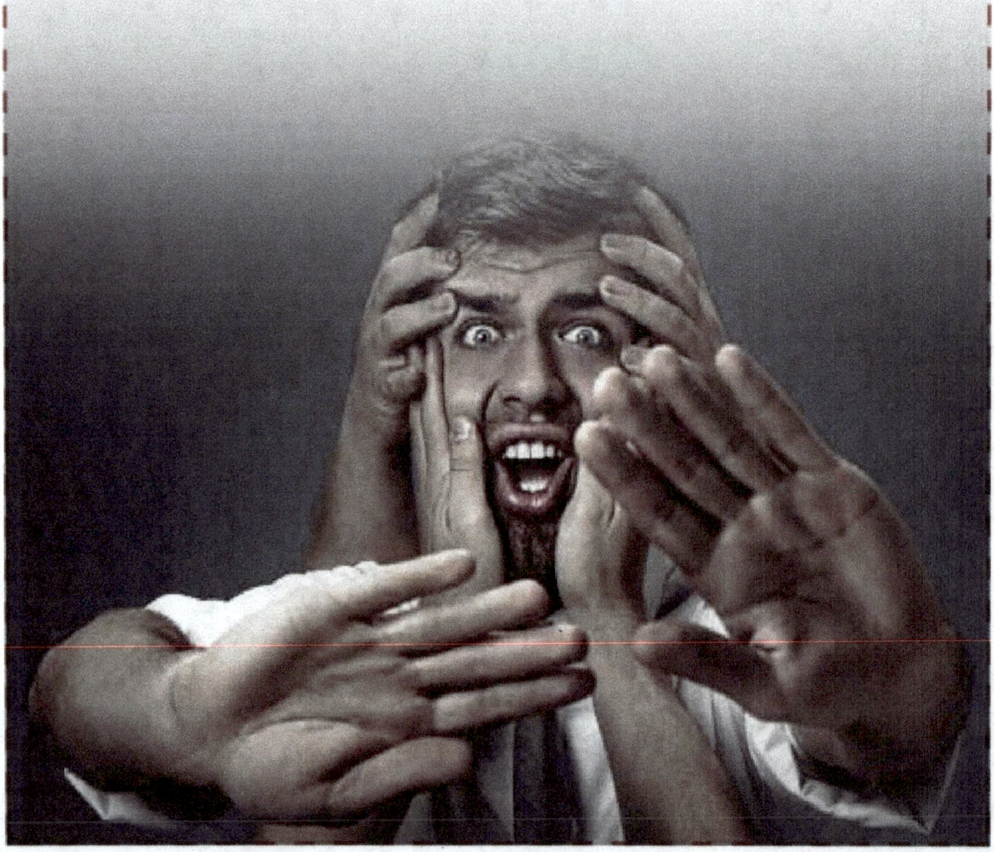

A strategic approach to defeat cancer

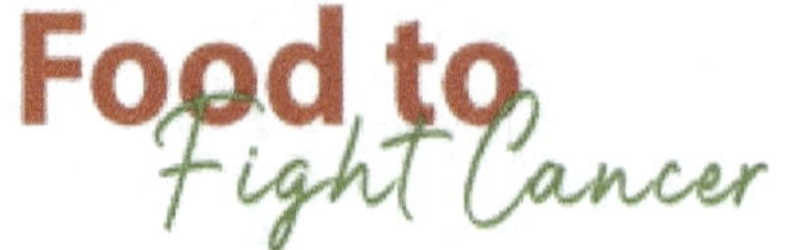

A strategic approach to defeat cancer

A basic strategy to fight cancer needs to include the following approaches:

1- Decrease exposure to carcinogens.

2- Enhance the ability of the liver to detoxify the toxins that aggravate **cancer** (Effective Liver Detoxification).

3- Fight the oxidative damage to our cells via the intake of sufficient antioxidants.

4- Improve our DNA repair mechanisms.

5- Adequate methylation of our DNA.

6- Enhancing the process of programmed cell death of **cancer** cells (apoptosis).

7- Improve the ability of our immune system so that it attacks and gets rid of the **cancer** cells.

8- Impede new vessel formation inside **cancer** cells (angiogenesis).

9- Inhibit the ability of the proteases that allow **cancer** cells to destroy the surrounding tissues and to spread to other areas.

10- Sufficient intake of nutritional compounds that can kill **cancer** cells.

11- Decreasing contributing negative health factors that may aggravate **cancer**, such as obesity, stress and psychological depression.

12-A positive attitude in the war against **cancer** (Yes, I can defeat it).

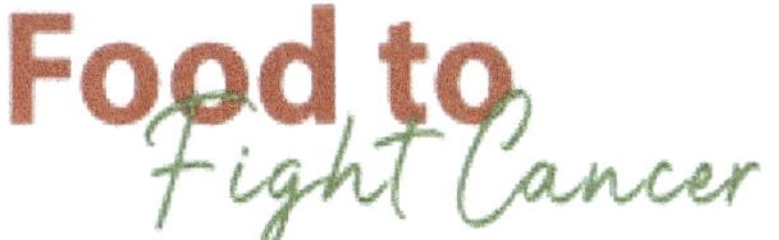

A strategic approach to defeat cancer

Carcinogenesis

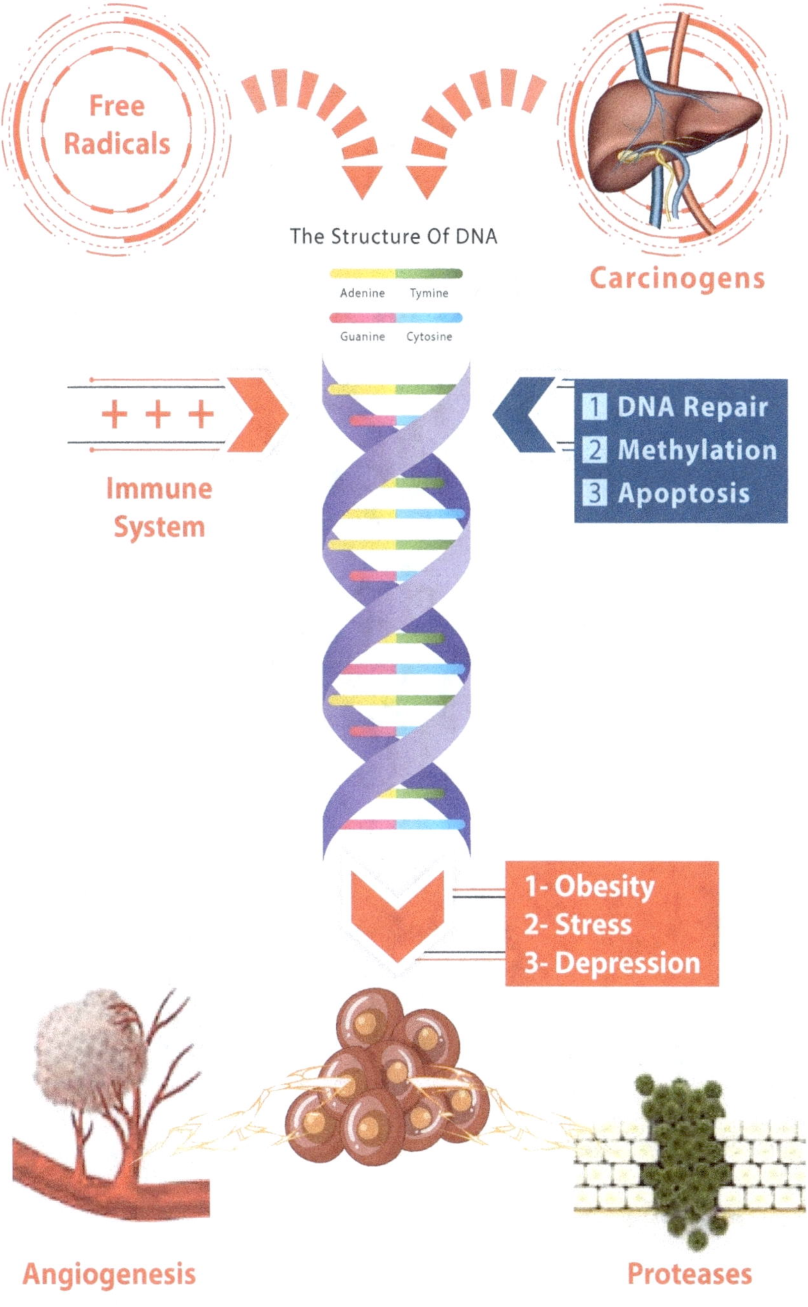

Specific steps that you can take to fight cancer

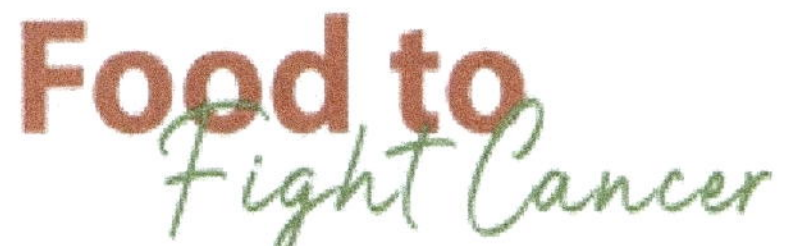

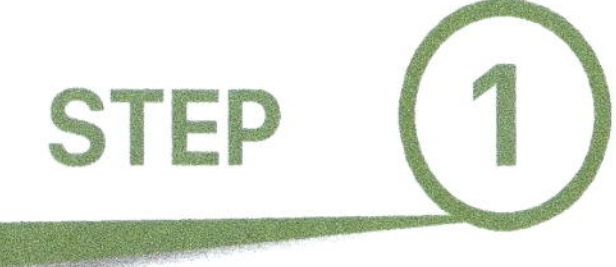

Believe that you can defeat it

One of the most important factors - if not the most important one - that can help you defeat cancer is to strongly believe that YOU can defeat it.

Thousands of cancer survivor stories have shown concrete evidence that YOU CAN DEFEAT IT, irrespective of its stage.

However, if you surrender to cancer and lose hope that you can defeat it, you may develop depression.

Depression can impair your immune system and reduce your body's ability to kill cancer cells, so it is important to try and stay positive.

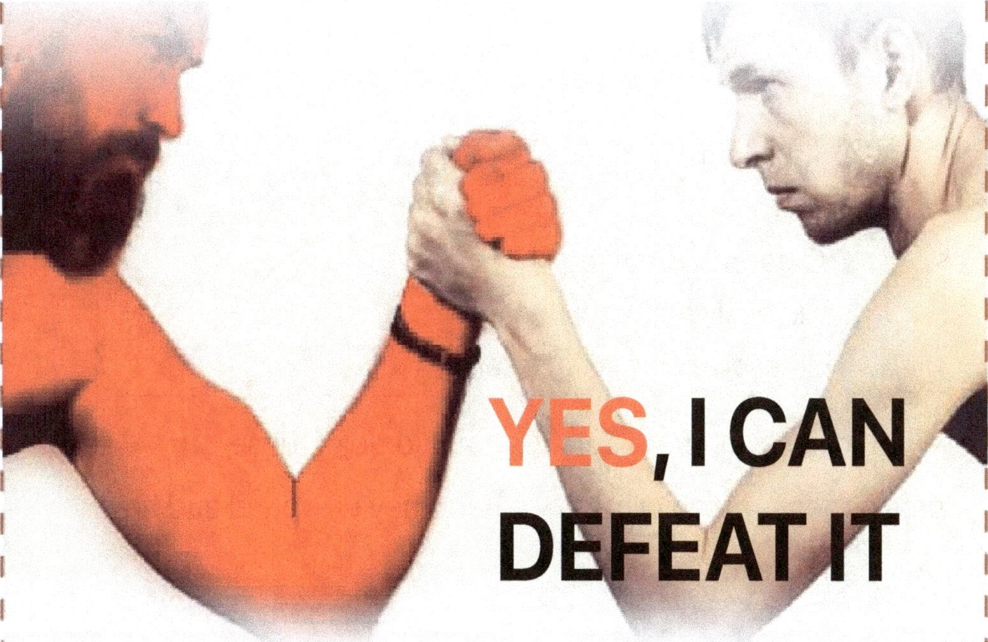

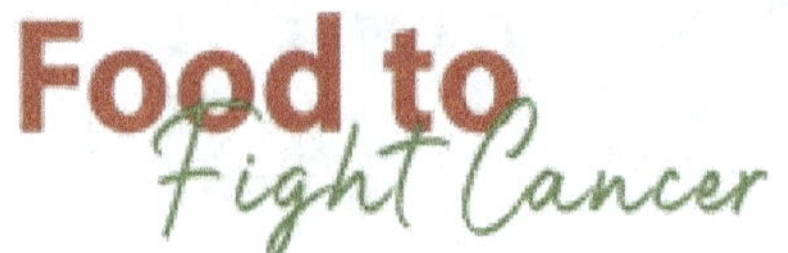

STEP 2

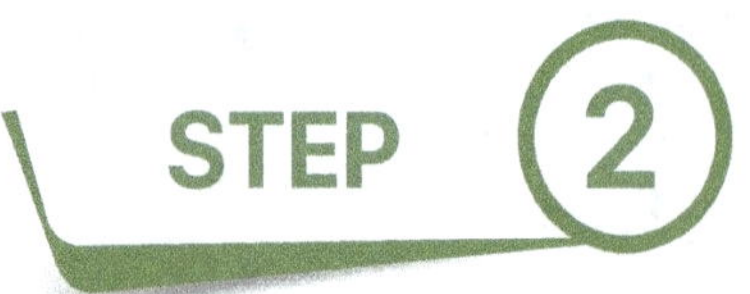

Decrease exposure to carcinogens

In general, it is better to avoid (or at least decrease) exposure to well known carcinogens.

As explained earlier, carcinogens are compounds that may damage the regulatory areas of our DNA or work via other molecular mechanisms to aggravate the cancerous process.

A list of well-known carcinogens and their sources is below:

1	Anti-Cancerous drugs
2	Polycyclic and Heterocyclic Aromatic Hydrocar bons
3	Vinyl chloride, Nickel, and Chromium
4	Insecticides & Fungicides
5	Nitrosamines
6	Aflatoxin
7	UVRs
8	Cigarette Smoking
9	Excessive alcohol intake
10	Excessive animal fat intake

What follows are more details about some of these carcinogens, which will show where they are found and how they can be avoided.

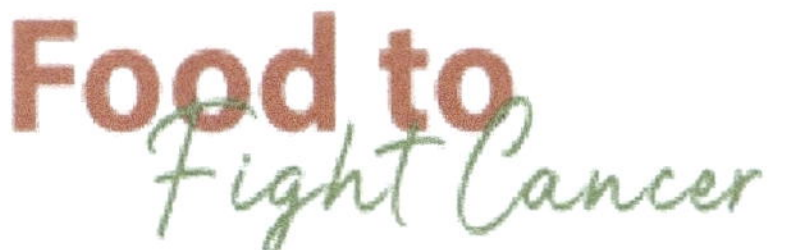
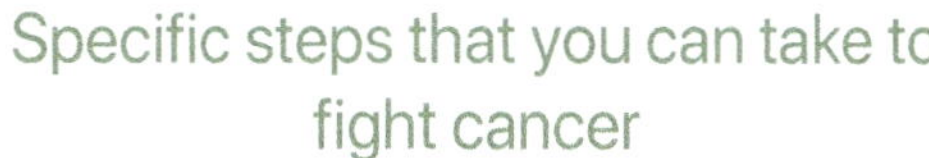

Food to *Fight Cancer*

Polycyclic aromatic hydrocarbons (PAHs) and heterocyclic amines (HCAs) are chemicals formed in meat, including beef, pork, fish or poultry, when they are cooked using high-temperature methods, such as pan frying or grilling directly over an open flame.

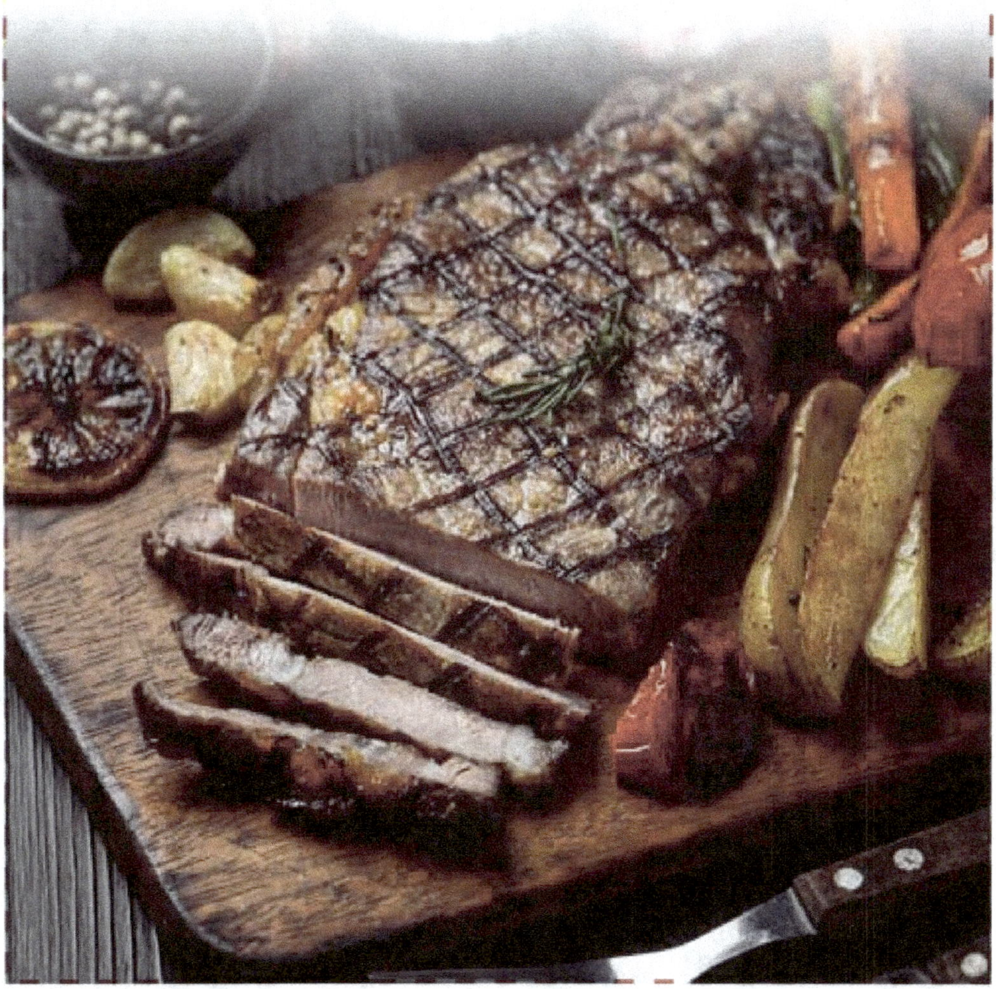

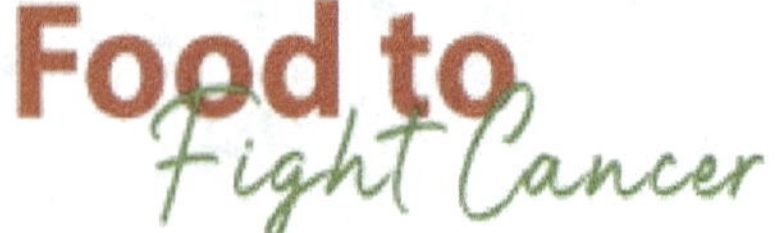

Food to Fight Cancer

Sources of nitrosamines include nitrite preserved food like luncheon meats, bacon or smoked fish.

It is important to note that **vitamin C** can inhibit the formation of such dangerous nitrosamine compounds in the gut.

It is advisable to avoid these compounds if possible.

Should you eat any of these foods, it is recommended that you should supplement them with some lemon, as lemon contains high levels of **vitamin C**.

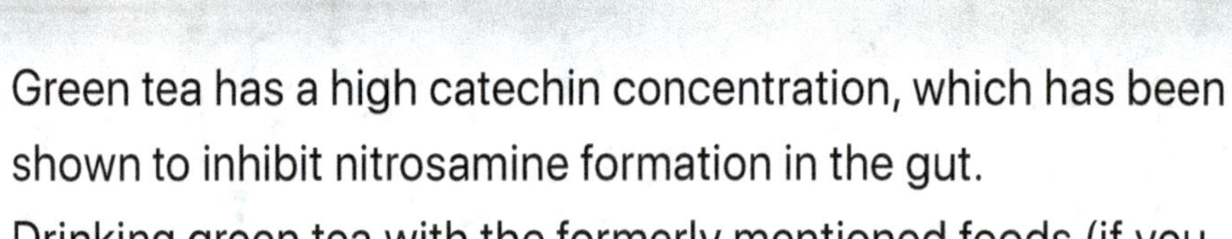

Green tea has a high catechin concentration, which has been shown to inhibit nitrosamine formation in the gut.

Drinking green tea with the formerly mentioned foods (if you can't altogether avoid eating them) can be very useful.

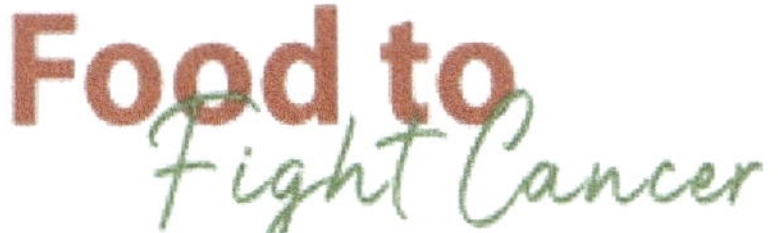

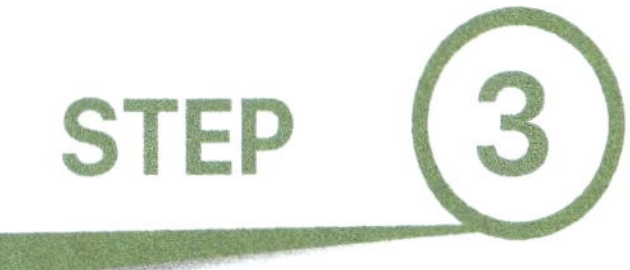

Effective liver detoxification

Detoxification refers to specific metabolic pathways that process unwanted chemicals for elimination.

Most of the detoxification process occurs in the liver.

Inside the liver cells there are sophisticated mechanisms to break down toxic substances.

Nearly every drug, artificial chemical, pesticide and hormone, is broken down (metabolized) by enzyme pathways inside the liver cells.

Inefficient removal of toxins by the body can result in the accumulation of several toxic compounds that may cause damage and mutations to our DNA, thus aggravating the cancerous process.

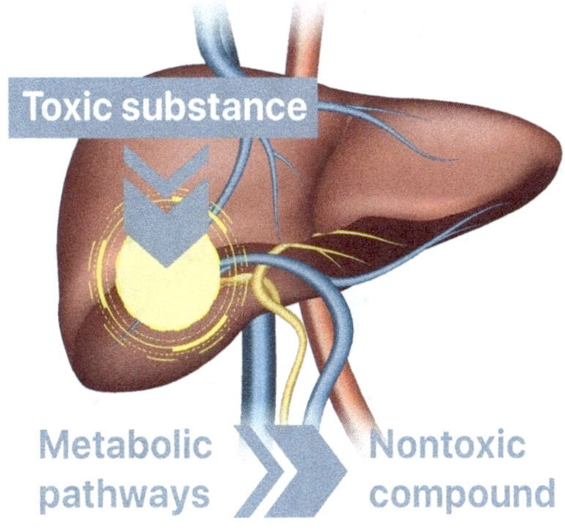

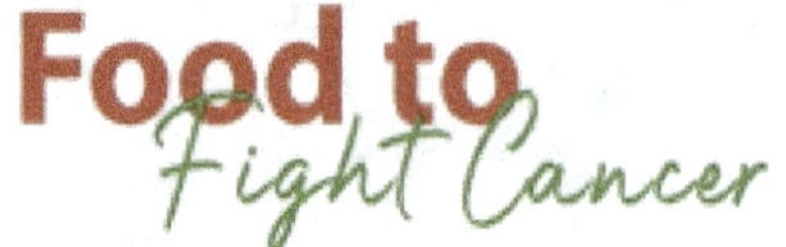

Glutathione plays a fundamental role in several metabolic and biochemical reactions in the detoxification process in our body and is thus considered to be the most powerful liver detoxifier and protector.

As we will see next, glutathione has multiple functions.

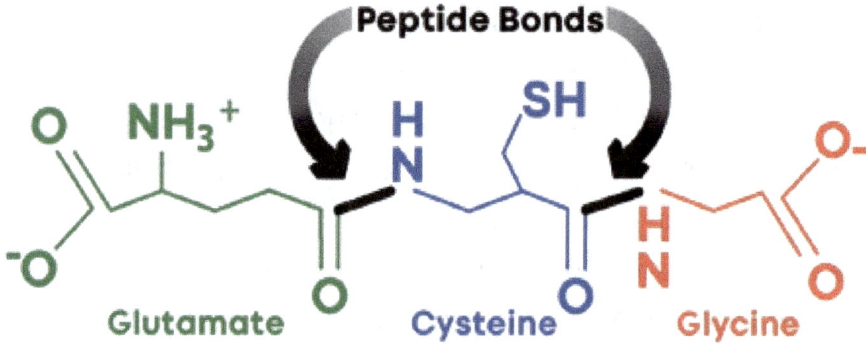

Glutathione- a powerful liver detoxifier- is formed of 3 amino acids: Glutamic acid , cysteine- and glycine

As the major antioxidant produced by the cells, glutathione participates directly in the neutralization of free radicals.

It also maintains antioxidants such as **vitamin C** and **E** in forms that can be used by the body.

Through direct conjugation, it detoxifies many foreign chemical compounds and carcinogens, both organic and inorganic, and also heavy metals such as mercury, lead and arsenic.

It is also critical for removing air pollutants such as volatile organic chemicals, and also many pesticides.

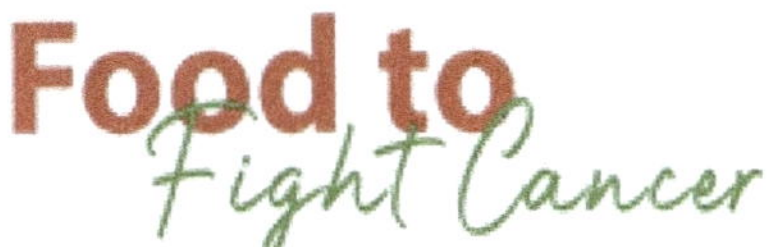

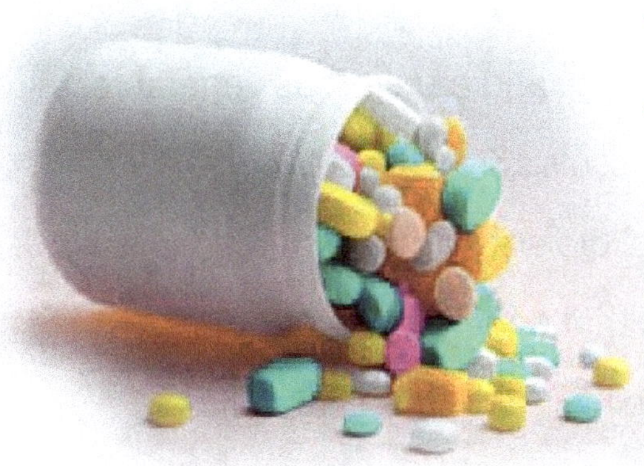

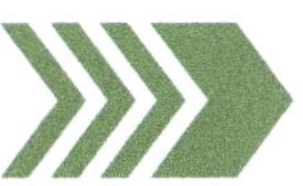
Neutralization of free radicals

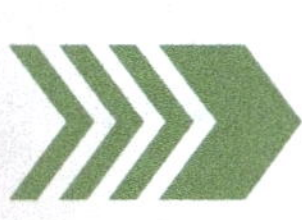
Maintains antioxidants such as vitamins C and E in active forms

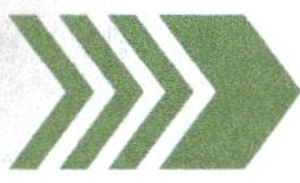
Detoxifies many foreign chemical compounds and carcinogens

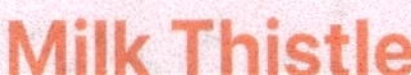

Milk Thistle

Herb stimulates glutathione activity and is the most commonly taken supplement for liver detoxification.

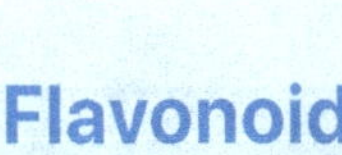

Flavonoids

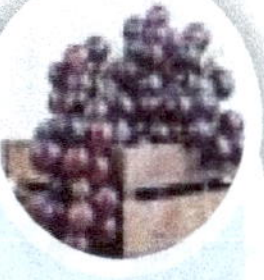

From red grapes and blueberries help regenerate depleted glutathione levels. Grape seed extract can be an excellent supplement.

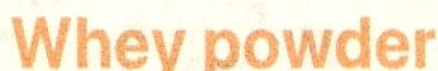

Selenium

is crucial for recycling glutathione and is regarded as an anticancer nutrient as a result. It is highest in brazil nuts and oysters and is also found in wholegrain products – especially those organically grown.

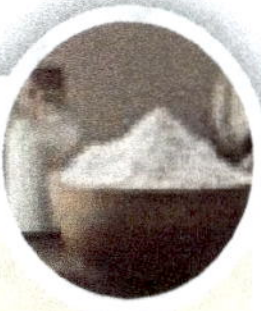

Whey powder

is a good source of cysteine, the critical amino acid needed for glutathione production.

Food to Fight Cancer

Green tea encourages liver detoxification, as does limonene oil, which can be found in the peel of citrus fruits.

Additionally, whey powder, eggs and cruciferous vegetables (e.g., broccoli, cabbage, Brussels sprouts, cauliflower), raw garlic, onions, leeks and shallots are all good sources of the natural sulphur compounds that enhance an important detoxification reaction in the liver, known as sulphation.

All of these foods can be considered to have a cleansing effect. Blending some of these compounds and drinking them as a juice can be very helpful in fighting **cancer**.

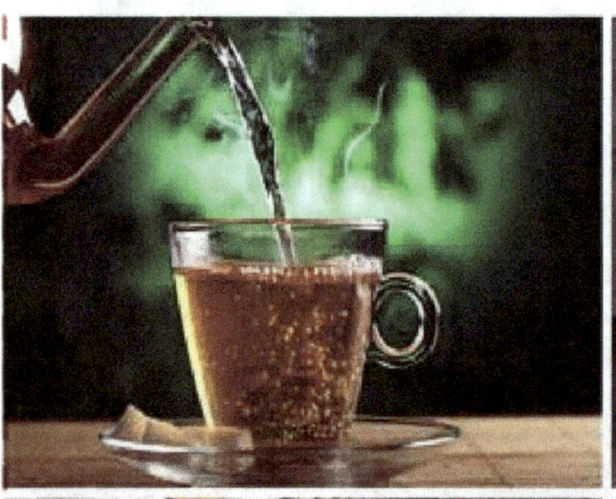
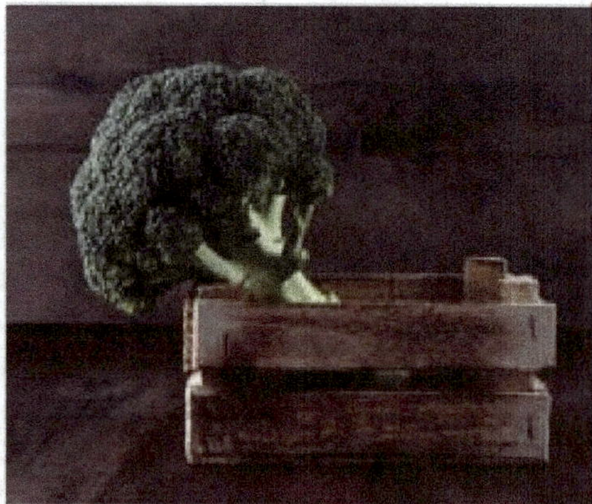
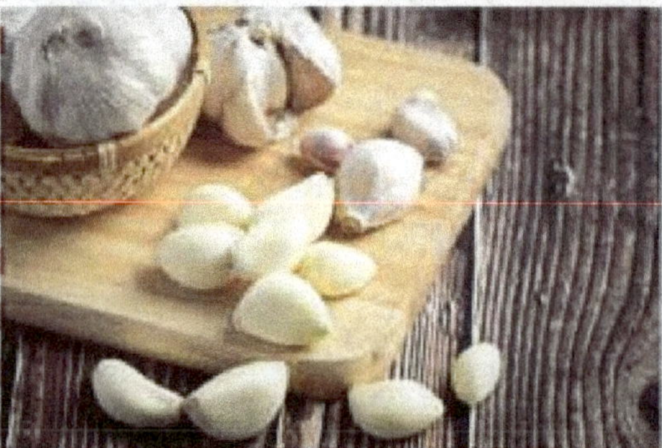
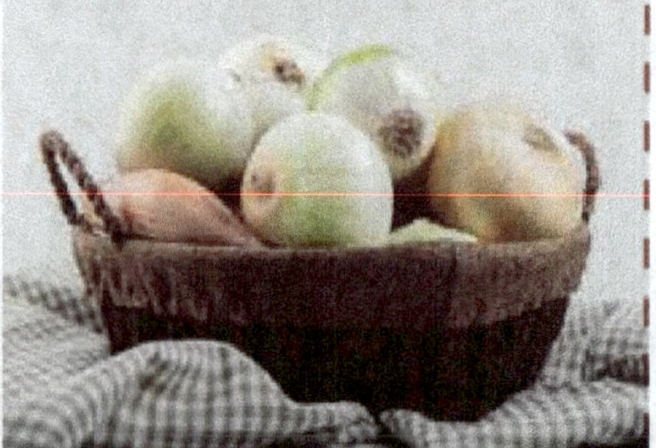

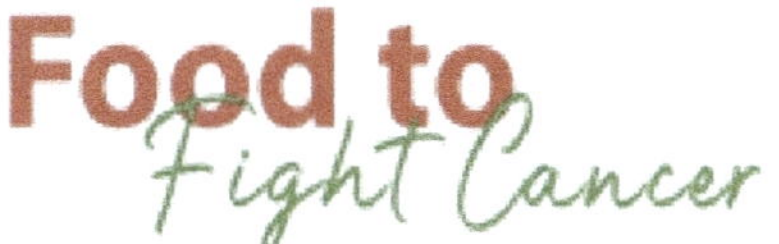

Food to
Fight Cancer

Curcumin, the compound that gives turmeric its yellow color, is particularly effective in regenerating glutathione after it has been oxidized.

This effect can be very useful in preventing certain types of **cancer**.

Curcumin has been found to inhibit carcinogens (such as benzopyrene, found in charcoal-grilled meat).

Additionally, it appears that curcumin exerts its anti-carcinogenic attributes by lowering the activation of carcinogens through its anti-oxidant properties.

At the same time, it increases detoxification by improving the active form of glutathione.

Curcumin can possibly help reduce the cancer-causing effects of tobacco.

Moreover, curcumin has also been shown to directly inhibit the growth of some **cancer** cells, particularly lung and bowel **cancer**.

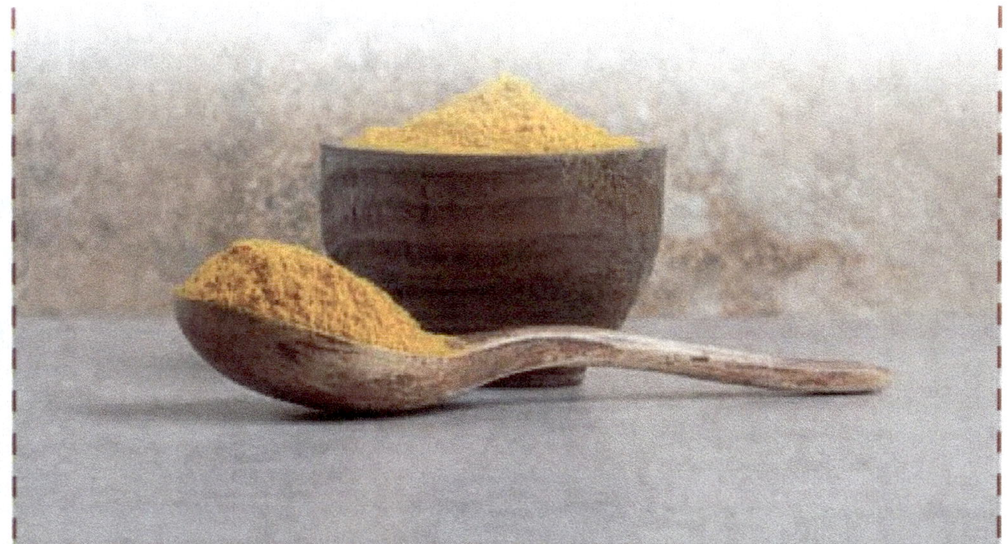

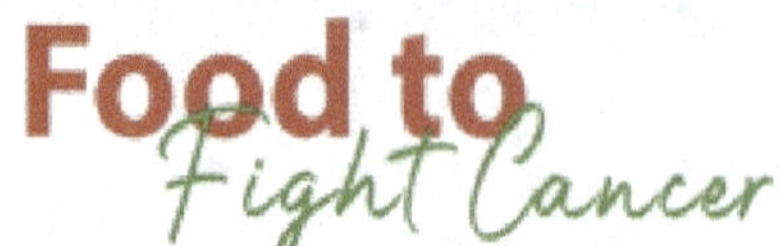

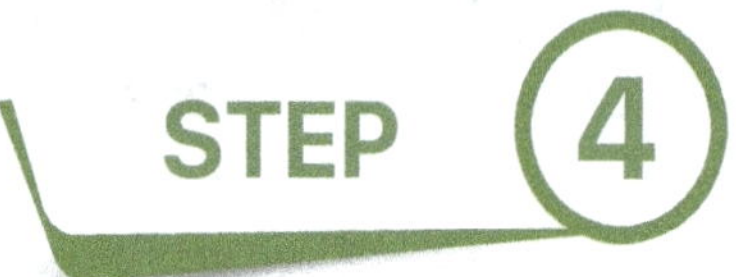

Have sufficient intake of antioxidants

Importance of Antioxidants

In addition to cancer, free radicals are involved in the development of many diseases such as atherosclerosis, inflammatory joint disease, asthma, diabetes, senile dementia and degenerative eye disease. Antioxidants can bind such free radicals in the body and may thus help us fight **cancer** and other diseases as well.

Sources of Antioxidants include

1- Carrots

2- Grapes

3- Blue berries

4- Fish

5- Tea

6- Whole grains

7- Beans

8- Nuts

9- Dark green vegetables

10- Sweet potatoes

- Beta-carotene
- Lutein
- Lycopene
- Selenium
- Vitamin A
- Vitamin C
- Vitamin E

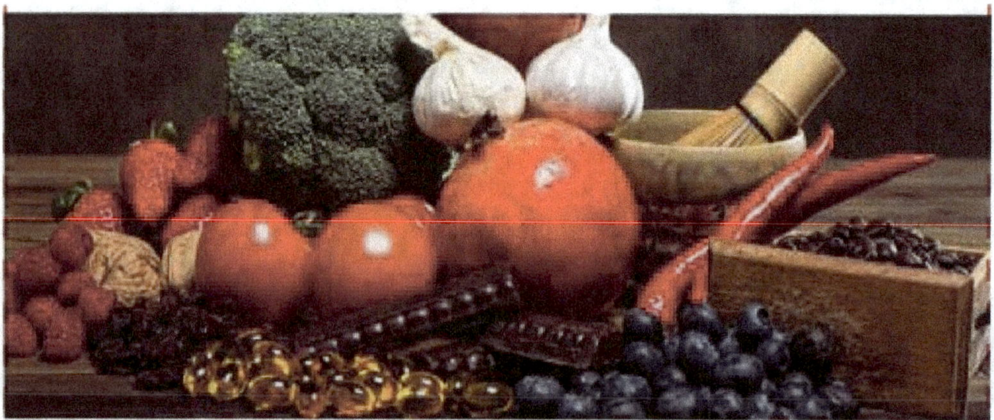

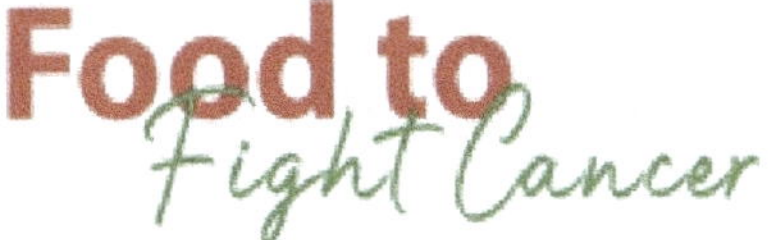

Vitamin C is a water-soluble vitamin. This means that the ability of your body to store it is limited.

We can get what we need from food, including citrus fruits, broccoli and tomatoes.

Results of some population-based studies suggest that eating foods rich in vitamin C may be associated with lower rates of **cancer**.

It is important to note that smoking cigarettes lowers the amount of vitamin C in the body, so smokers are at a higher risk of vitamin C deficiency than non-smokers.

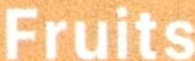

Fruits

1- Oranges
2- Papaya
3- Kiwi fruit
4- Strawberries
5- Pine apples

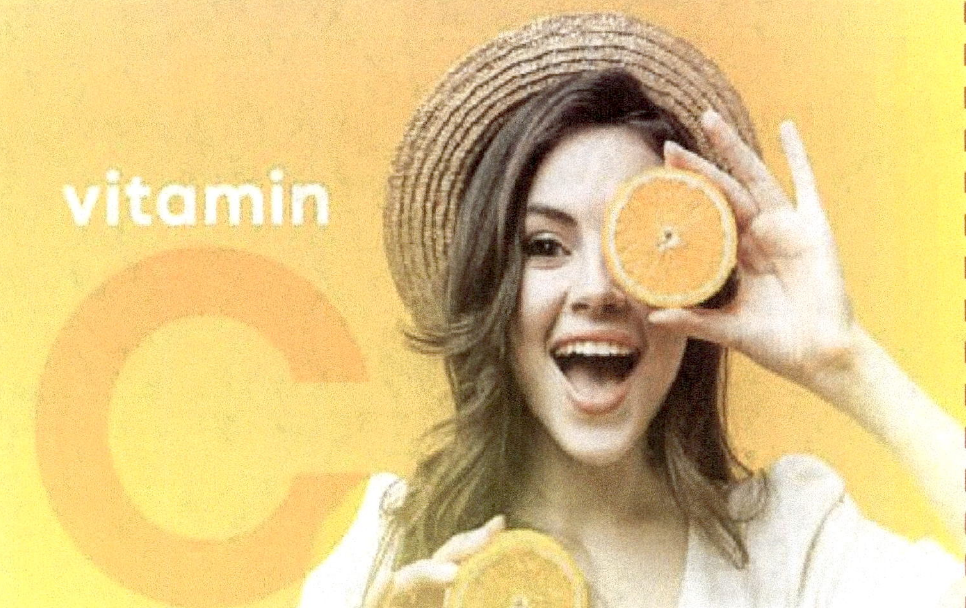

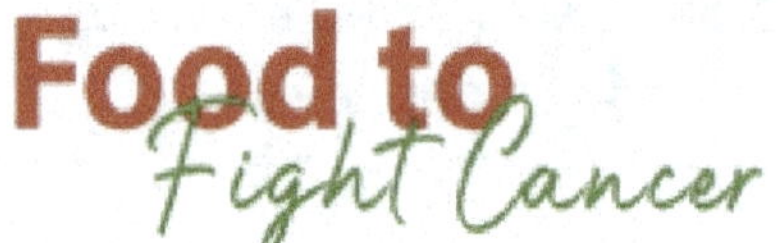

Vitamin E is a powerful, fat-soluble antioxidant that helps protect cell membranes against damage caused by free radicals.

Vitamin E encompasses a group of eight compounds, called tocopherols and tocotrienols.

The best way to get the daily requirement of vitamin E is by eating food sources which contain it, such as:

1- Vegetable oils (such as wheat germ, sunflower, safflower, corn, and soybean oils)

2- Nuts (such as almonds, peanuts, and hazelnuts/filberts)

3- Seeds (such as sunflower seeds)

4- Green leafy vegetables (such as spinach)

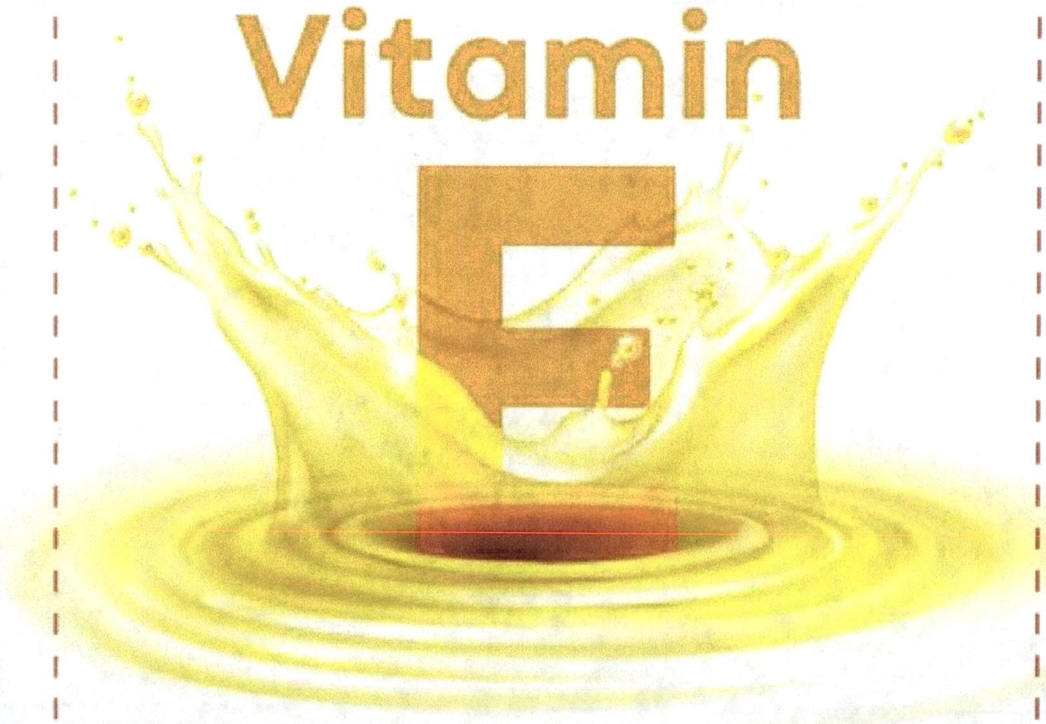

Food to *Fight Cancer*

Specific steps that you can take to fight cancer

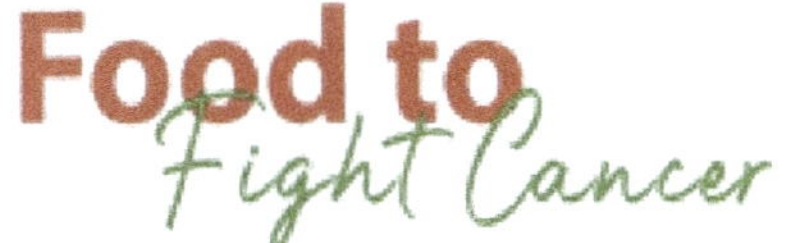

Beta-carotene is a carotenoid.

Carotenoids are naturally occurring pigments found in plants and are largely responsible for the vibrant colors of some fruits and vegetables.

Once ingested, beta-carotene is either converted into vitamin A (retinol), which the body can use in a variety of ways, or it acts as an antioxidant to help protect cells from the damaging effects of harmful free radicals.

Sources of Beta-carotene

1- Carrots
2- Sweet potatoes
3- Pumpkins
4- Spinach
5- Beet root
6- Kale

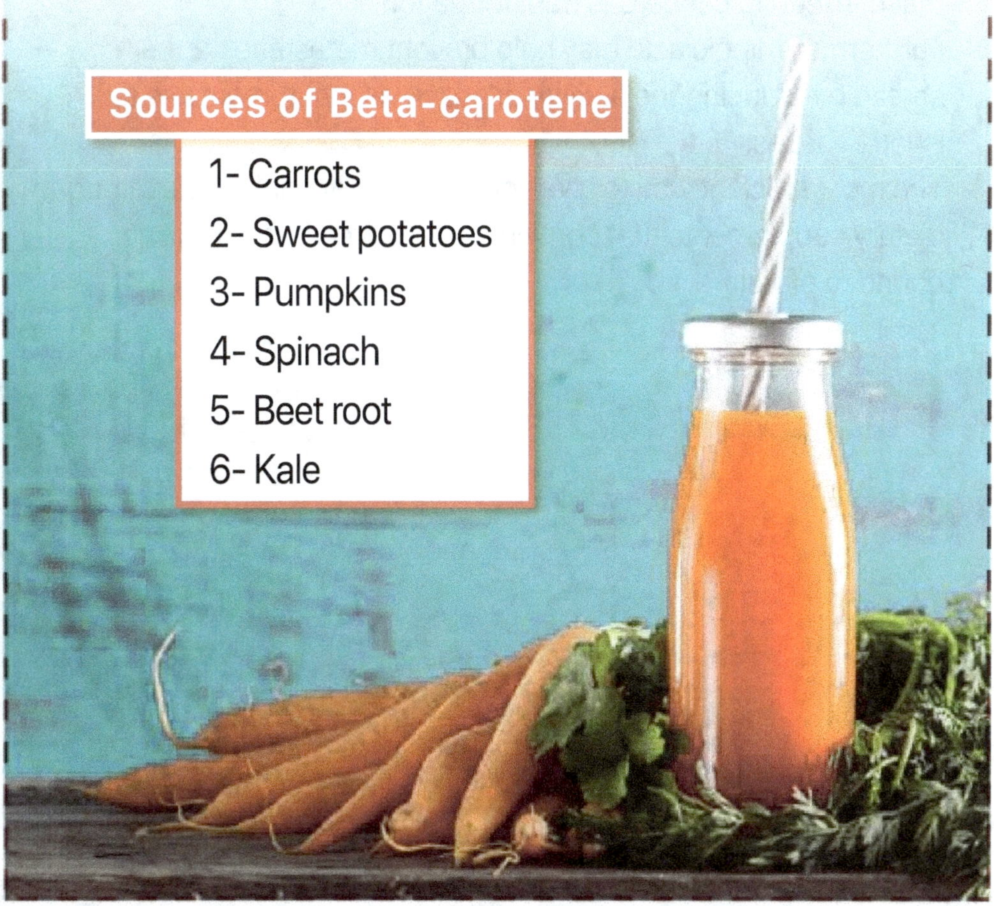

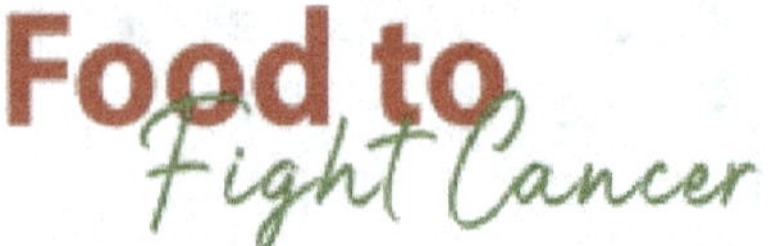

Food to
Fight Cancer

Lipoic acid (also known as a-lipoic acid or ALA) has several anti-inflammatory features that may assist in fighting **cancer**. These features allow lipoic acid to intervene at multiple points in the chain of carcinogenesis.

Preliminary research indicates that lipoic acid can stop the reproductive cycle of **cancer** cells, slowing or stopping tumor growth.

Additionally, lipoic acid may help induce the programmed cell death that is the body's natural control mechanism for weeding out nascent **cancers**.

Lipoic acid also protects against chemical-induced DNA damage that can lead to cancerous transformation.

Furthermore, lipoic acid may help prevent metastatic **cancer** spread by reducing the activity of enzymes that tumors use to invade tissues.

The most efficient way to give your body additional ALA is through dietary supplements that contain ALA in a free form that is not bound to protein.

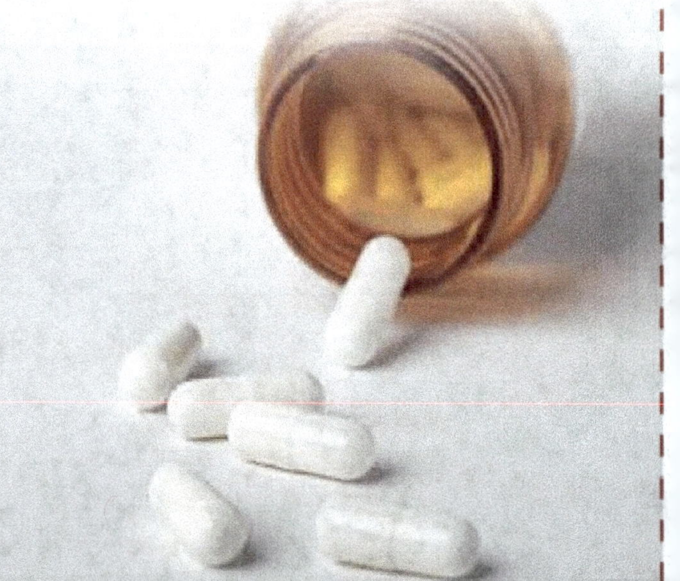

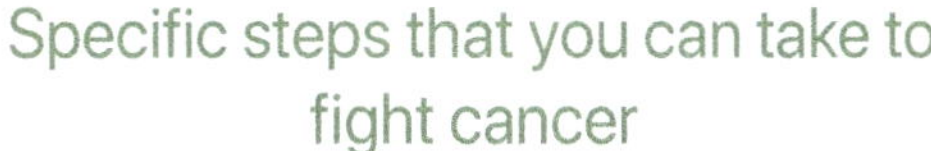

Food to *Fight Cancer*

Specific steps that you can take to fight cancer

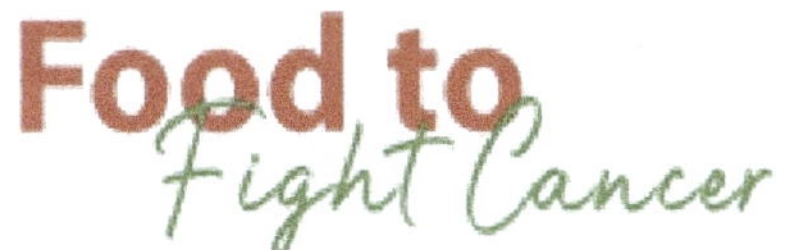

Lycopene is a red biological compounds found predominantly in tomatoes and tomato products, such as ketchup and tomato sauce. In addition to its anti-oxidant properties, lycopene can inhibit human **cancer** cell growth by interfering with growth factor receptors that aggravate the proliferation of **cancer** cells. Additionally, lycopene may enhance the activity of (or up-regulate) a gene called connexin 43.

The activation of this gene by lycopene may improve cellular communications that inhibit the growth of **cancer** cells.

Such anti-**cancer** effects of lycopene may particularly affect prostate, breast and stomach **cancers**.

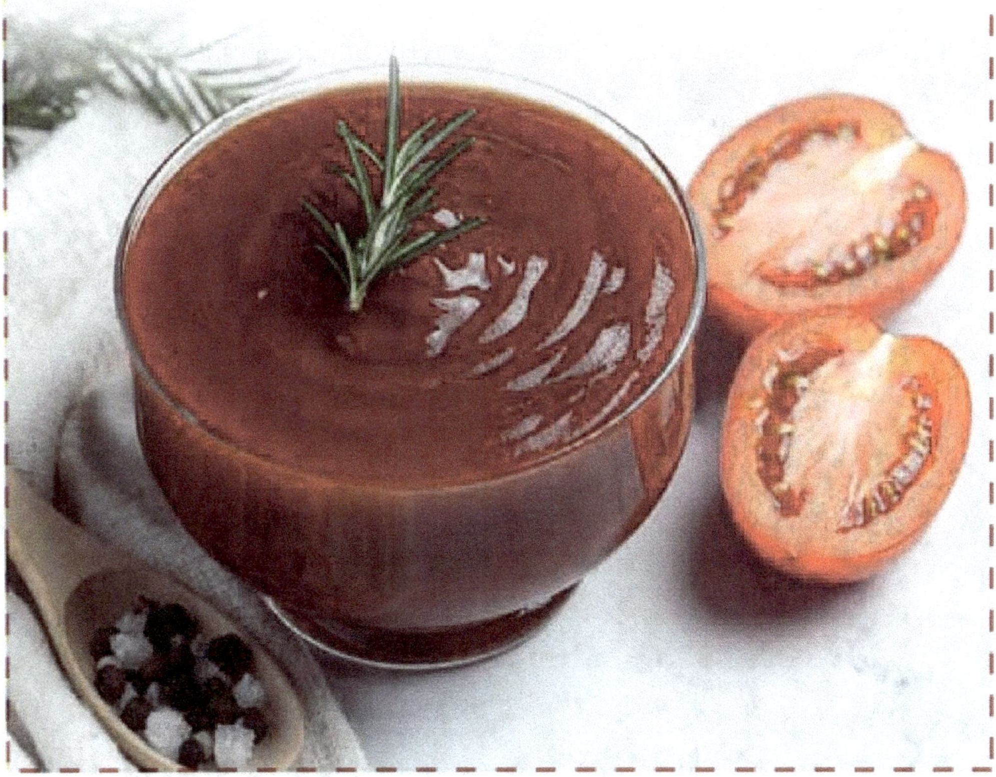

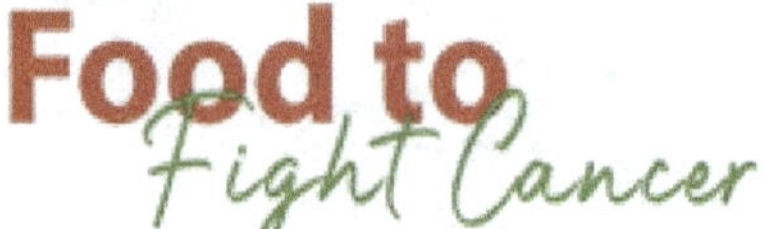

Coenzyme Q10 is a natural antioxidant synthesized by the body.

It is found in many foods and is also available as a supplement.

Interest in coenzyme Q10 as a possible treatment for **cancer**

began when it was found that some **cancer** patients had a lower

than normal amount of it in their blood.

More recent studies have identified probable mechanisms by

which CoQ10 may help slow tumor growth.

Some of these mechanisms include improving the ability of the

immune cells to fight **cancer**, suppression of new vessel formation

inside **cancer** cells (angiogenesis) and reduction of inflammatory

markers that may facilitate **cancer** cell propagation.

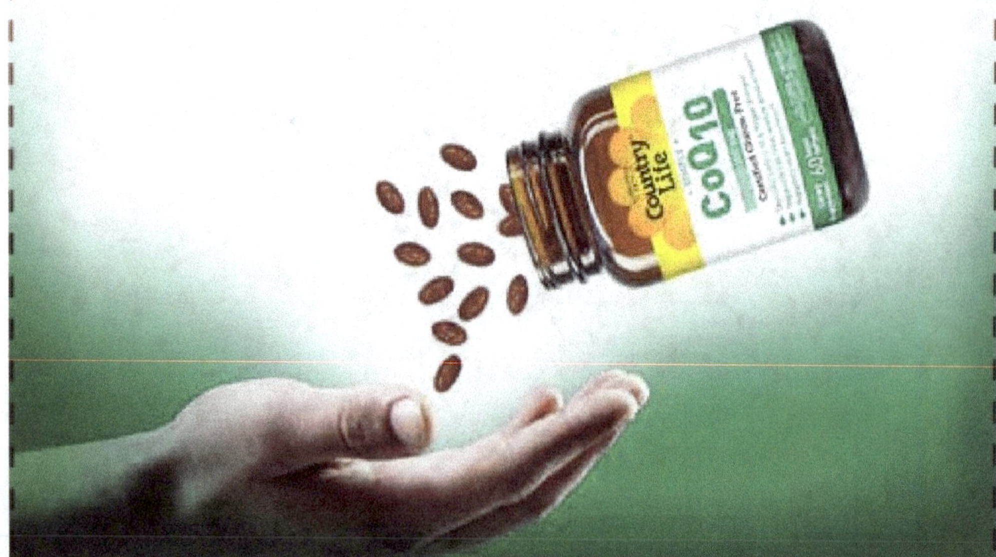

Food to Fight Cancer

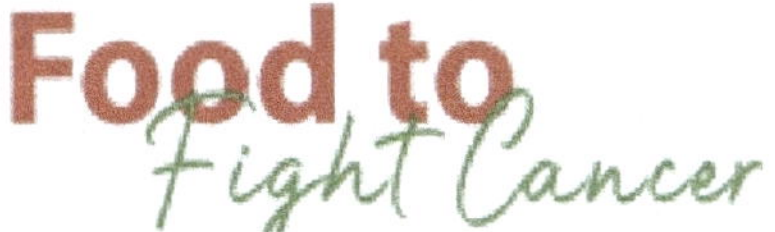

Flavonoids are one of the largest nutrient families known to humans, and include over 5,000 already-identified family members.

Some of the best-known flavonoids include quercetin, kaempferol, catechins and anthocyanidins.

This nutrient group is most famous for its antioxidant and anti-inflammatory health benefits.

They are abundant in apples, onions, tomatoes, parsley, celery, oranges, peaches, bananas, strawberries and blueberries.

Flavonoids exert anti-**cancer** properties as they:

1 - Fight free radicals in our body

2 - Affect cellular communication pathways, preventing the abnormal cell proliferation integral to the cancerous process

3 - Enhance programmed cell death (apoptosis), which can kill **cancer** cells when they are formed in the body

4 - Inhibit the process of angiogenesis (new vessel formation) in **cancer** cells.

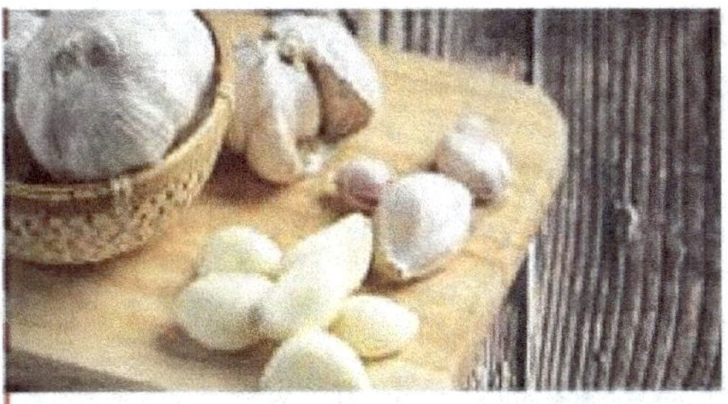
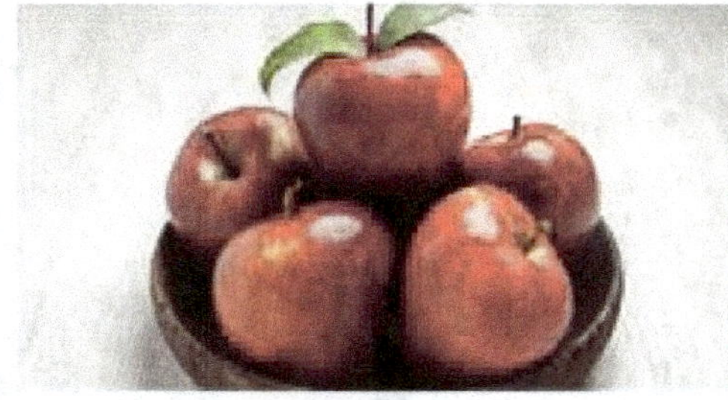
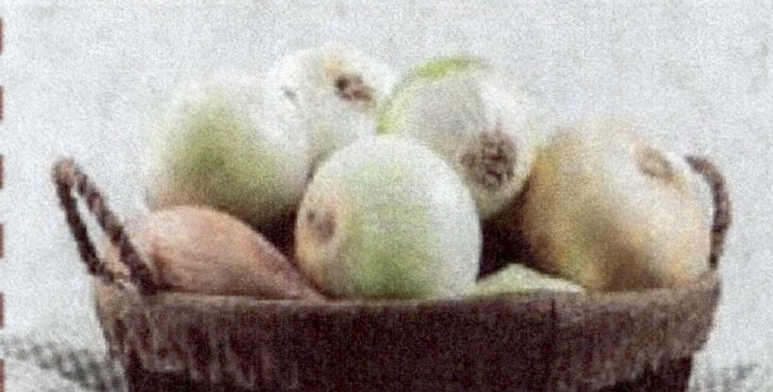
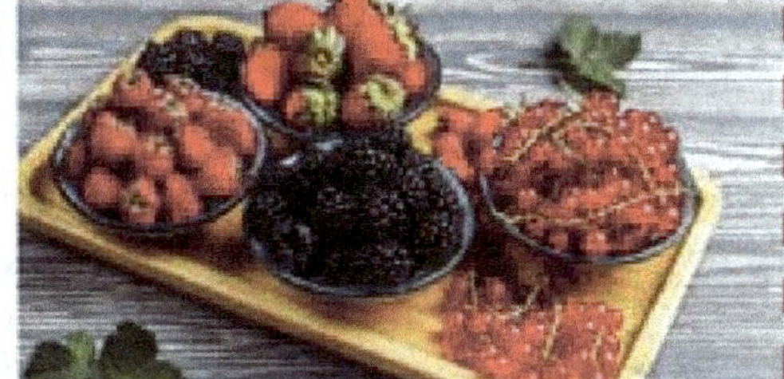

Food to *Fight Cancer*

Specific steps that you can take to fight cancer

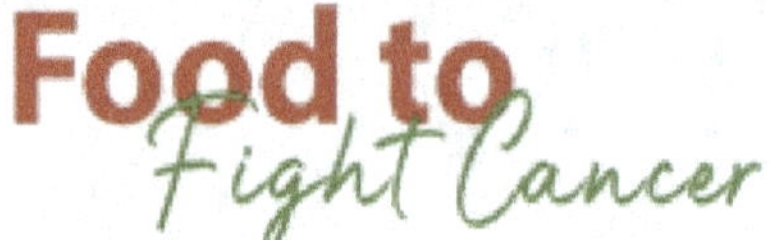

Resveratrol, a potent antioxidant found in a number of plants, including red grape skins, pomegranate, raw cacao, peanuts, and berries, is known to have a number of beneficial health effects. The highest concentration of resveratrol is found in red wine. Resveratrol has the ability to deeply penetrate the center of a cell's nucleus, allowing the DNA to repair free radical damage that might otherwise contribute to cancerous growth.

Furthermore, resveratrol's anti-inflammatory properties help prevent certain enzymes from forming that trigger tumor development.

It also helps cut down cell reproduction, which helps reduce the number of cell divisions that could contribute to the progression of **cancer** cell growth.

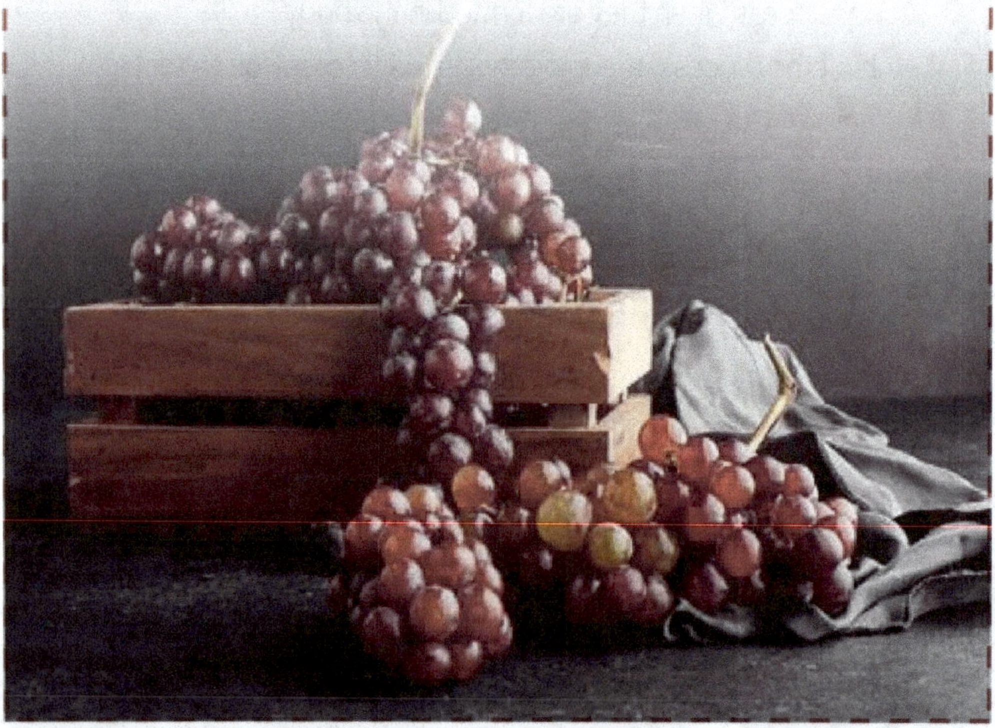

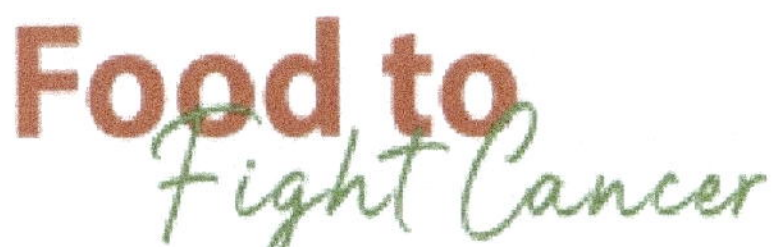

Food to Fight Cancer

STEP 5

Improve DNA repair

Even moderate consumption of alcohol may have an adverse effect on your DNA, as it induces oxidative DNA damage.

Specific examples of DNA - damaging molecules that are produced in the body as a result of alcohol consumption include reactive oxygen species, lipid peroxidation products and acetaldehyde.

Cigarette smoke can also cause DNA single strand damage in human cells.

One of the major constituents in cigarette smoke, hydroquinone, may be important for mediating smoke-induced DNA damage.

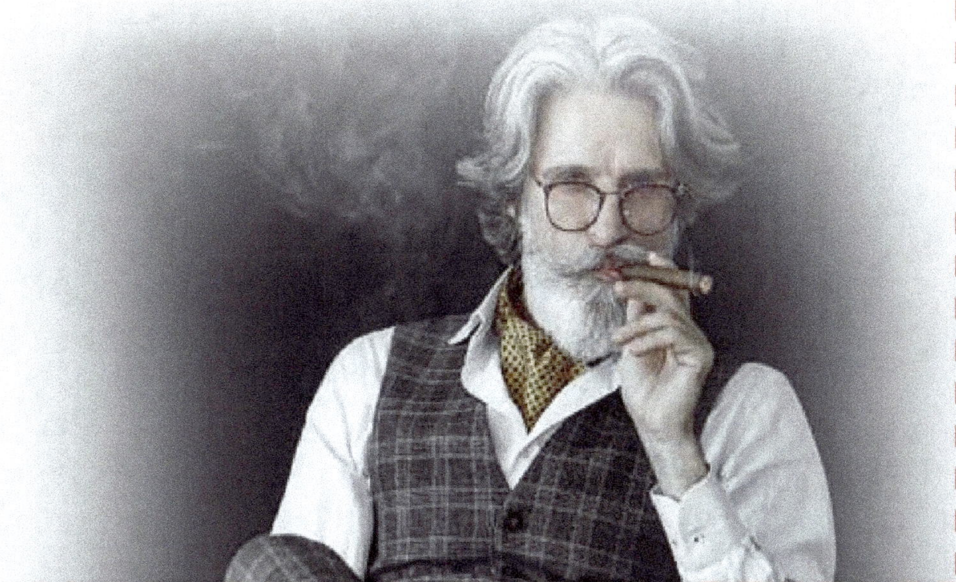

Food to
Fight Cancer

It is during sleep that cellular and DNA repair can take place.

Melatonin, a hormone that is produced by the pineal gland during sleep, may enhance DNA repair capacity by affecting several key genes involved in DNA damage responsive pathways.

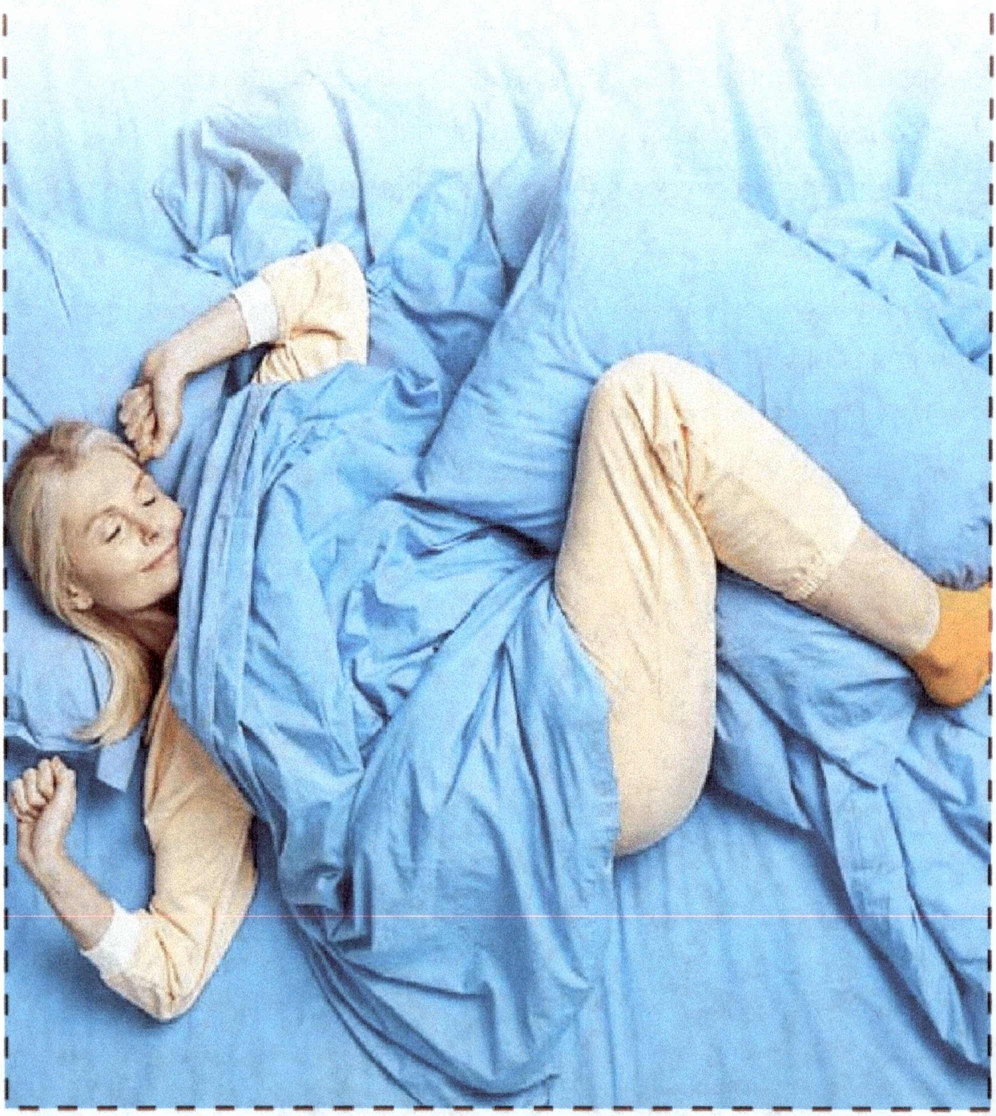

Food to *Fight Cancer*

Specific steps that you can take to fight cancer

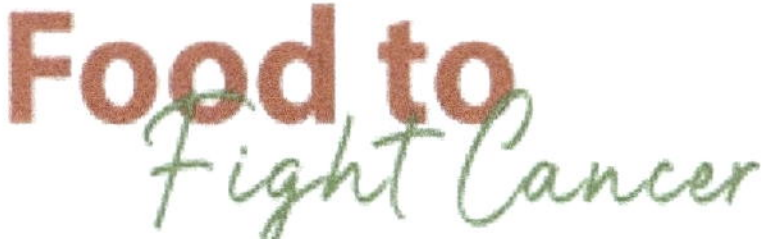

Engage in regular moderate exercise. Some studies show that regular exercise improves DNA repair in skeletal muscles and liver cells and reduces oxidative
damage done to the DNA in the liver.
Exercise also seems to enhance selective enzymes involved in de-toxification of
certain **cancer**-producing agents.
Additionally, moderate exercise can alter biological processes that contribute to the progression of **cancer**.

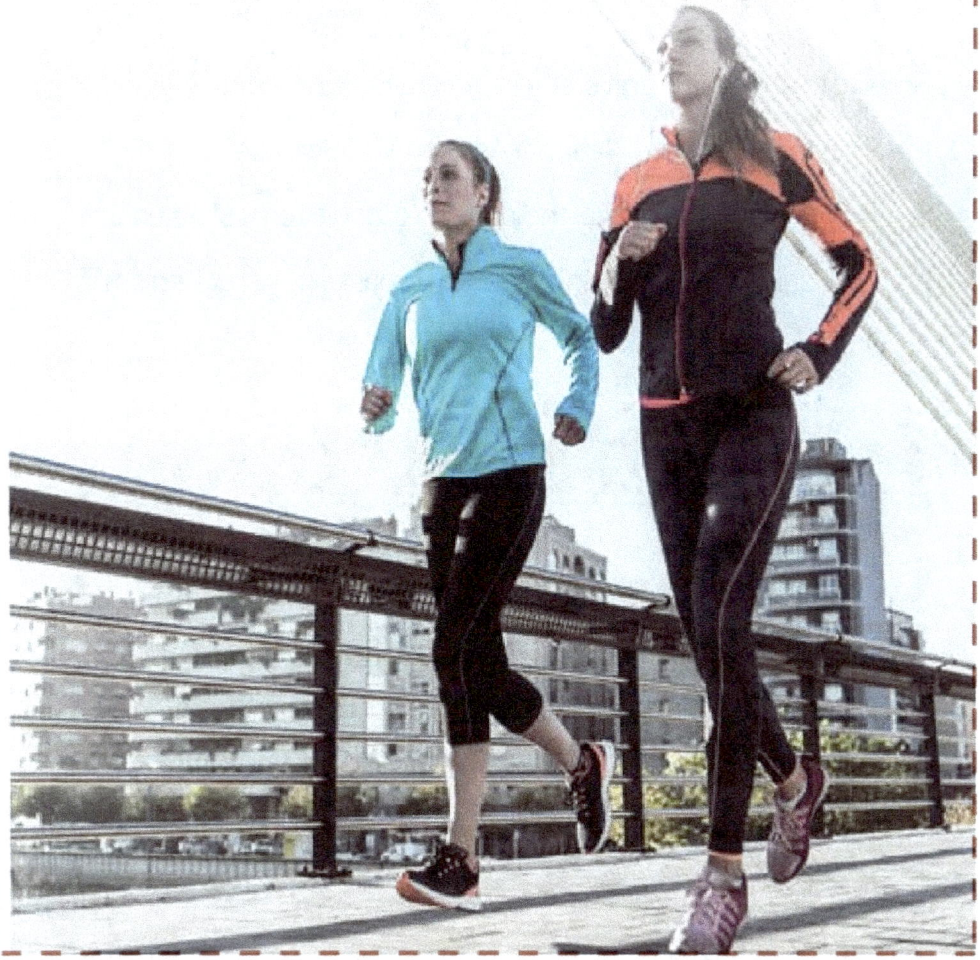

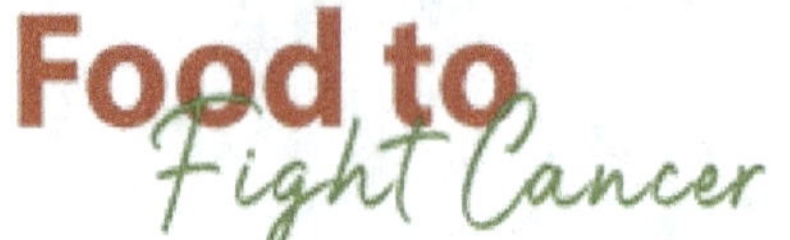

There is growing evidence that vitamin D selectively causes cell death in cancerous cells by interacting with copper ions. Additionally, it also increases the level of an endogenous protein, cystatin D, which possesses anti-tumor and anti-metastatic properties.

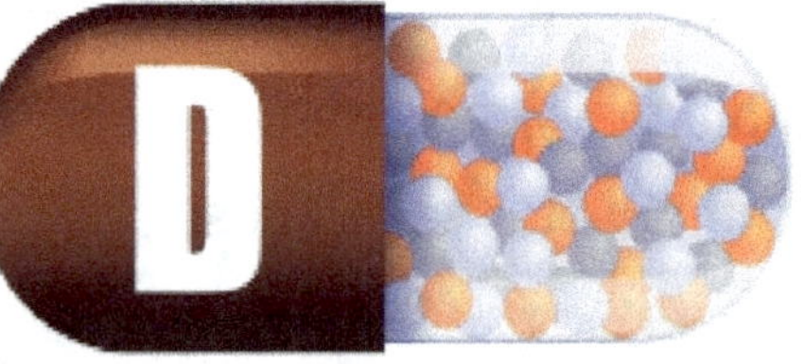

Scientists at Indiana University in Indianapolis reported in the Proceedings of the National Academy of Sciences that high levels of selenomethionine, the primary organic form of selenium, prompts cells in culture to initiate DNA repair, a key mechanism in fighting **cancer**.

Some of the best sources of selenium in our diet are listed below:

1- Brazil Nuts
2- Sunflower Seeds
3- Fish (tuna, halibut, sardines, flounder, salmon)
4- Shellfish (oysters, mussels, shrimp, clams, scallops)
5- Eggs

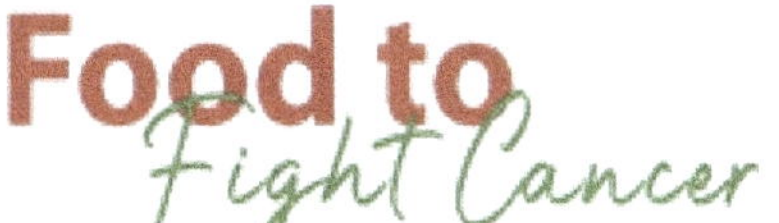

Kiwi fruit is also known to significantly increase the rate of DNA repair when three are eaten daily.

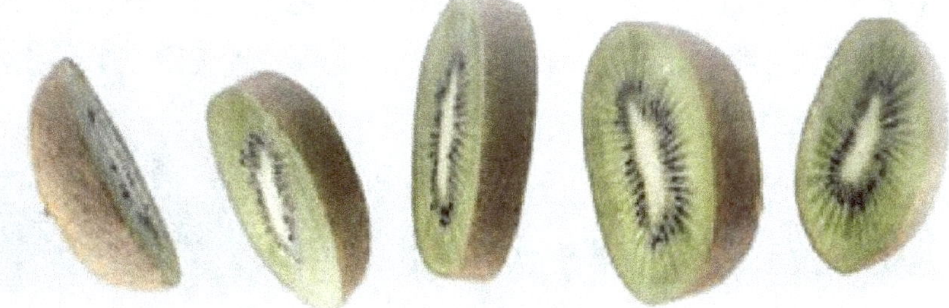

Citrus fruits and **cooked tomatoes** contain naringenin, which stimulates DNA repair in some **cancer** cells.

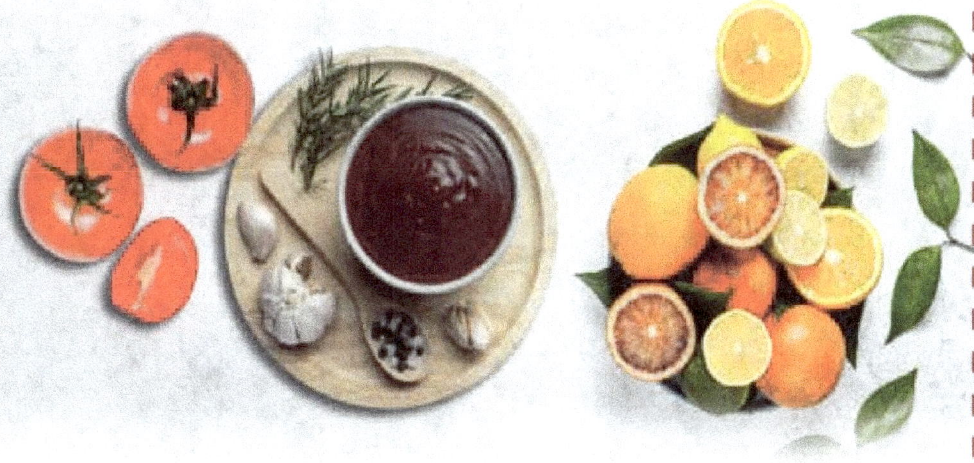

Phytic acid found in whole grains also promotes DNA repair.

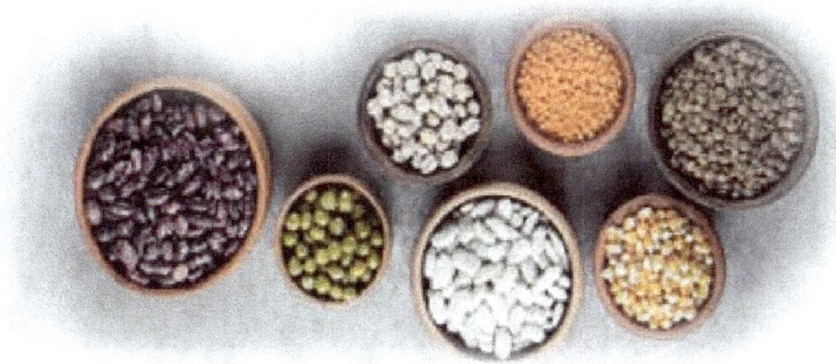

Food to Fight Cancer

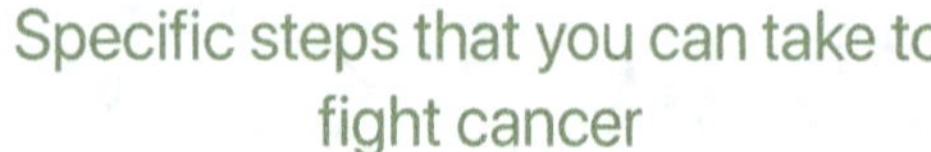

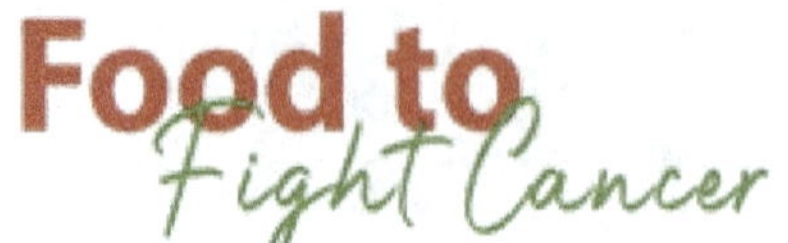

In a study published in the British Journal of **Cancer** (published by the research journal Nature), the researchers show that in laboratory tests, a compound called indole-3-carinol (I3C), found in broccoli, cauliflower and cabbage, can increase the levels of BRCA1 and BRCA2 proteins that repair damaged DNA.

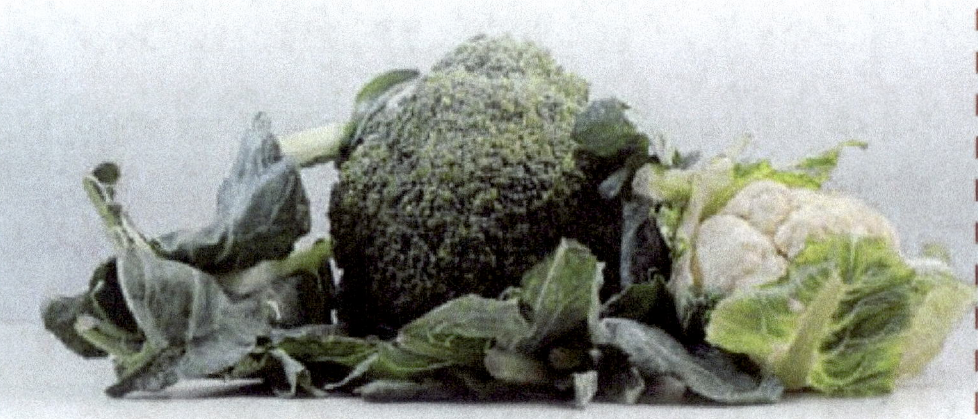

A deficiency in zinc impairs DNA repair.

Eating whole grains, leafy greens and sprouted legumes help to provide the body with zinc.

Oysters are considered one of the richest dietary sources for zinc.

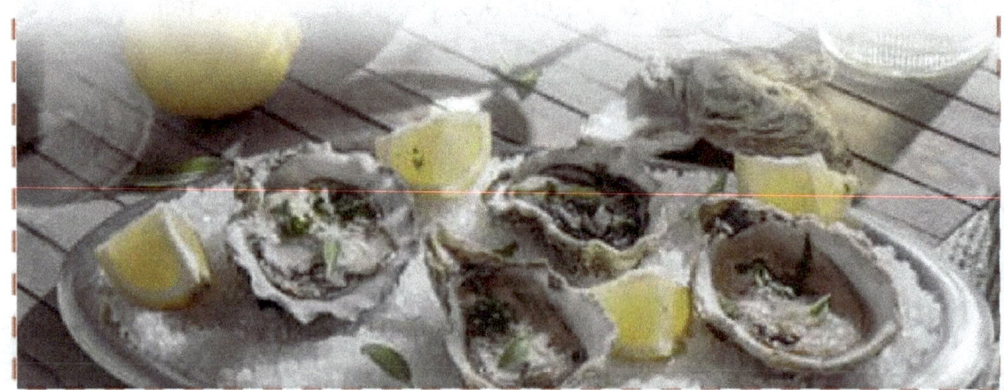

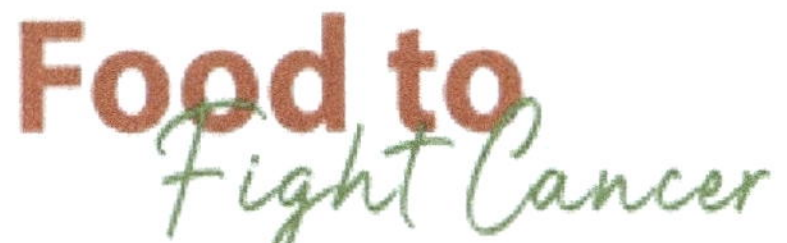

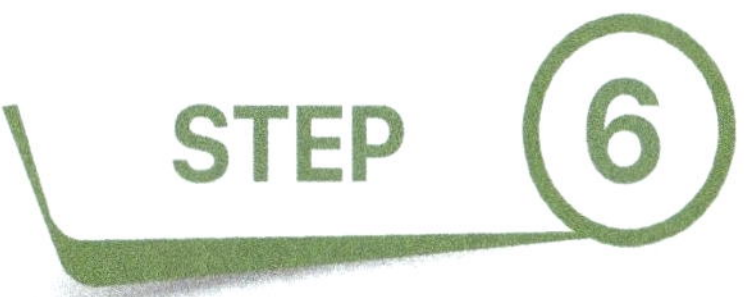

Adequate methylation of DNA

As explained earlier, DNA methylation plays an essential role in maintaining cellular function, and changes in the methylation patterns of our DNA may contribute to the development of **cancer**. Nutrients that play a role in the process of methylation of our DNA include folate, vitamin B12, vitamin B6, methionine and choline. Deficiency of these dietary factors may decrease S-Adenosyl Methionine, which is a key player in the methylation process of our DNA.

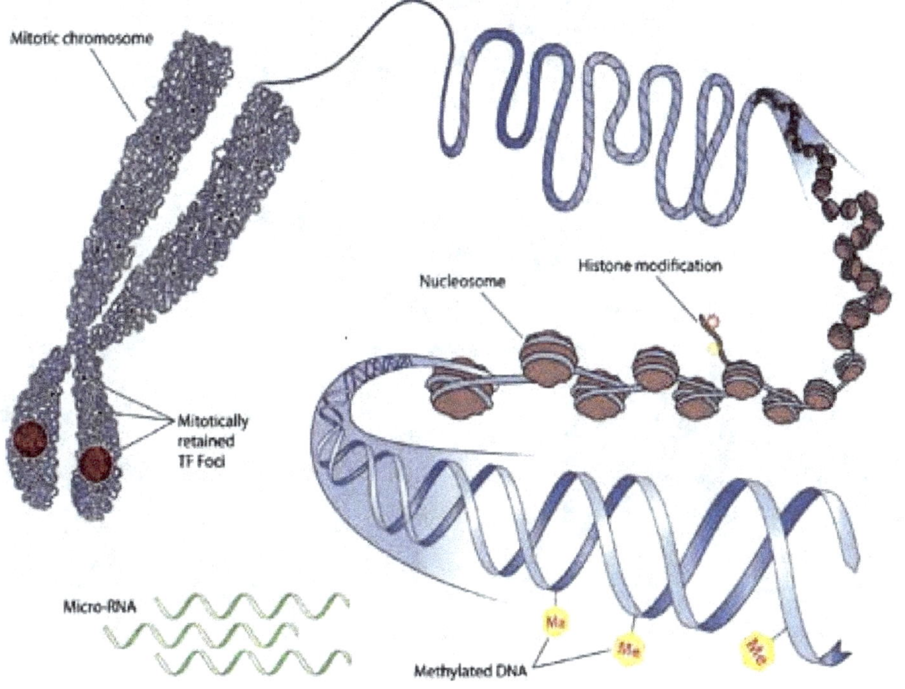

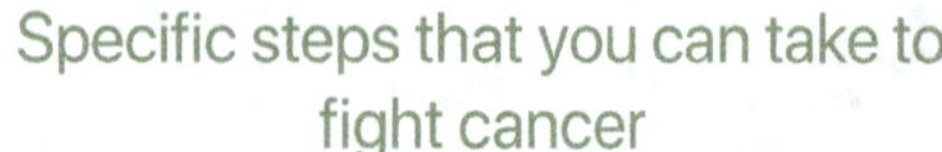

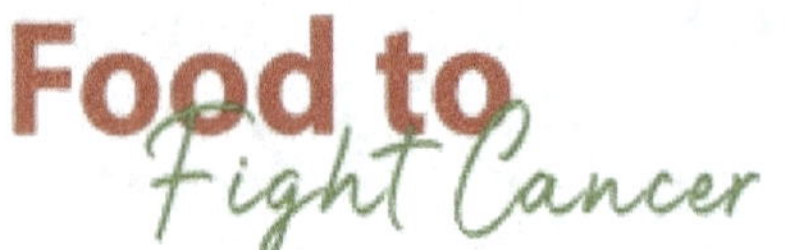

Food to Fight Cancer

Folic acid is important for proper DNA functions in our bodies:

Folic acid is water-soluble. Water-soluble vitamins dissolve in water. Excess amounts of the vitamin leave the body through the urine.

That means your body does not store sufficient amounts of folic acid and you need a continuous supply of the vitamin in the foods you eat.

Foods that are rich in folic acid include beans, asparagus, lentils, lettuce and avocado.

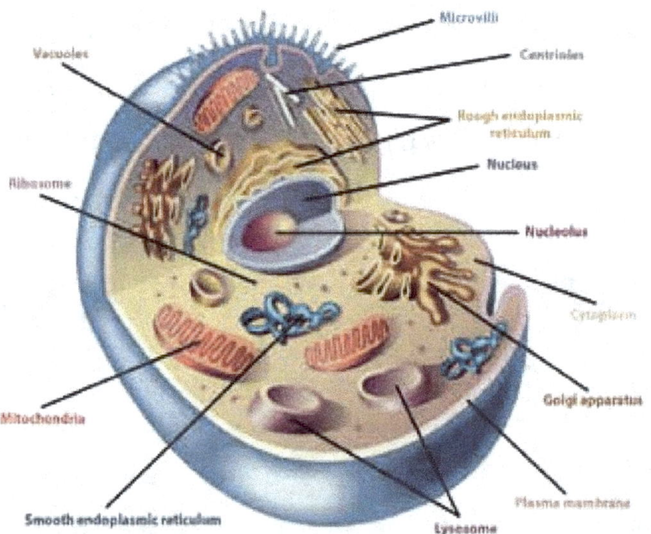

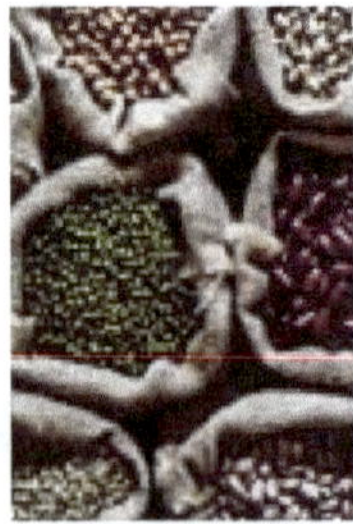

Beans

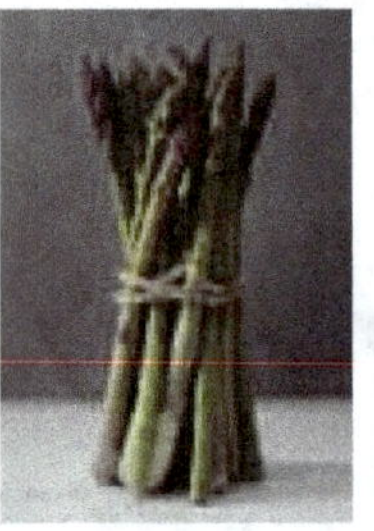

Asparagus

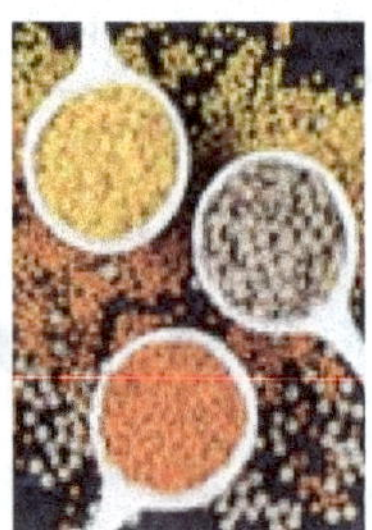

Lentils

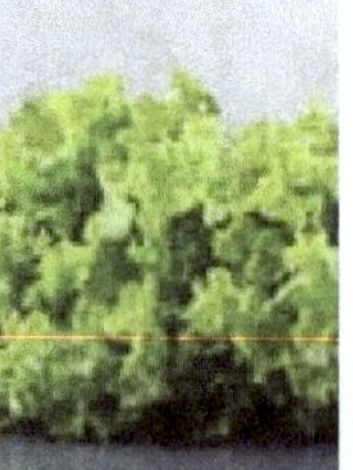

Lettuce

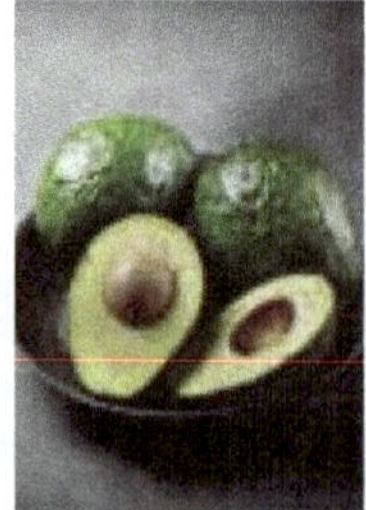

Avocado

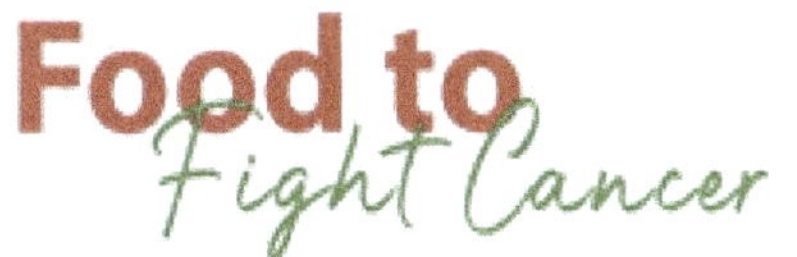

Vitamin B12 is a water-soluble vitamin that is naturally present in several foods (especially animal sources).

Vitamin B12 is important for DNA synthesis and ensures structural stability of important regions of the chromosomes.

As a methyl-donor, it participates in the metabolic pathways that leads to and plays a critical role in DNA methylation.

Low dietary consumption of **B12** results in respectively low serum levels, which induce alterations in DNA synthesis.

Thus, deficiency of **B12** may lead to DNA damage and aggravate cancer formation.

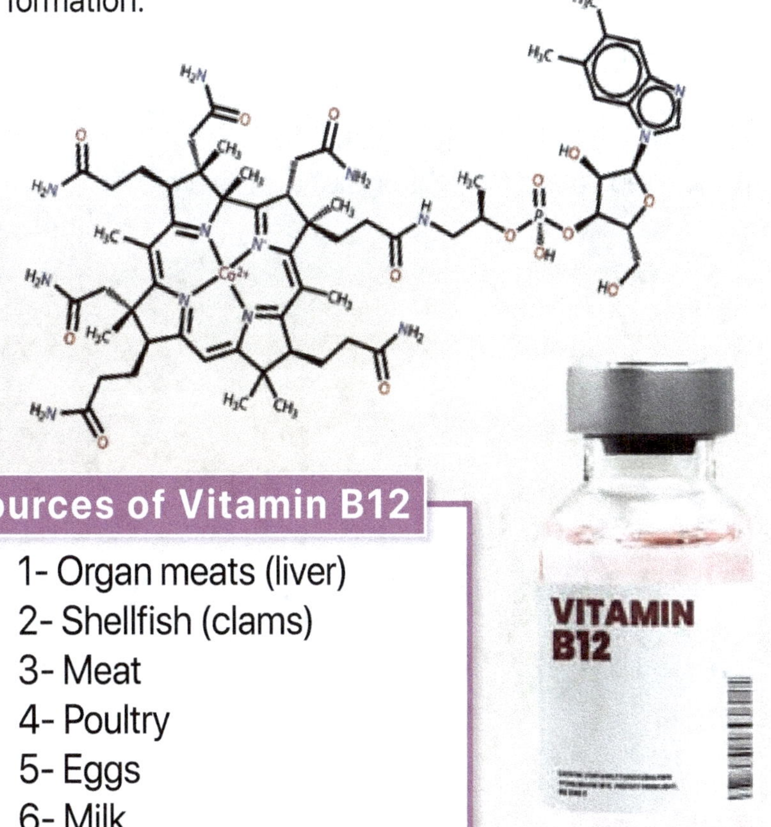

Sources of Vitamin B12

1- Organ meats (liver)
2- Shellfish (clams)
3- Meat
4- Poultry
5- Eggs
6- Milk

Food to
Fight Cancer

A global DNA hypomethylation might activate oncogenes in our cells to initiate **cancer**.

S-Adenosylmethionine (SAM) serves as a major methyl donor in the process of DNA methylation.

This may assist in suppressing **cancer** cells.

There is scientific evidence that SAM treatment inhibits cell growth in gastric **cancer** cells and colon **cancer** cells, and the inhibition efficiency was significantly higher than that in the normal cells.

It is possible that SAM can effectively inhibit the tumor growth by reversing the DNA hypo-methylation on promoters of oncogenes, thus down-regulating (or decreasing) their expression.

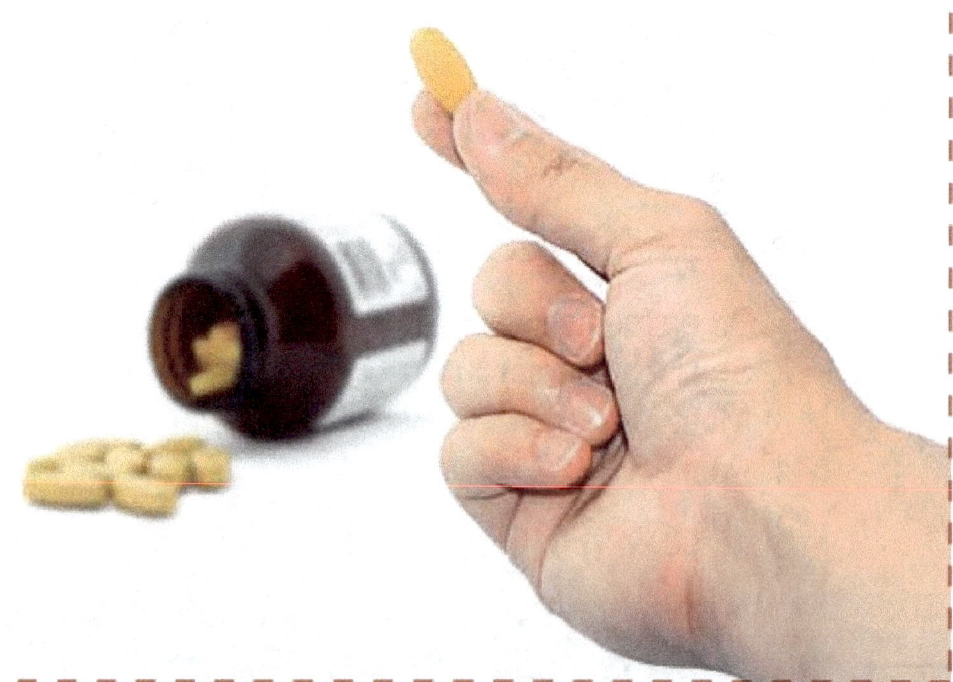

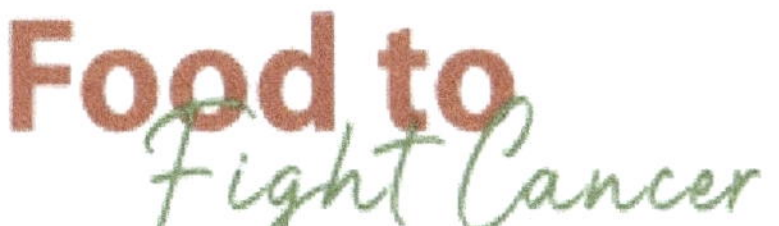

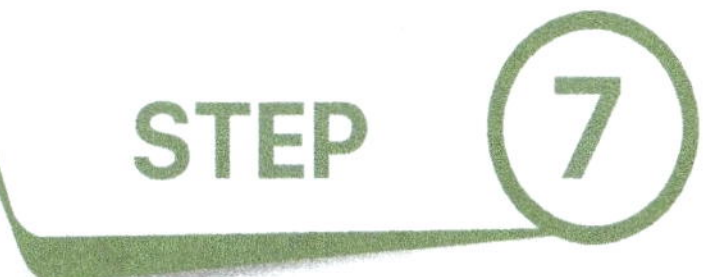

Enhancing apoptosis

Ginger originated in South-East Asia and is used in many countries as a spice and condiment to add flavor to food.

Besides this, ginger has also been used in traditional herbal medicine.

The bioactive molecules of ginger, like gingerols, have shown antioxidant activity in various modules.

Additionally, some constituents isolated from ginger affect cell proliferation and induce apoptosis, or programmed cell death.

These features explain why ginger has anti-cancer effects.

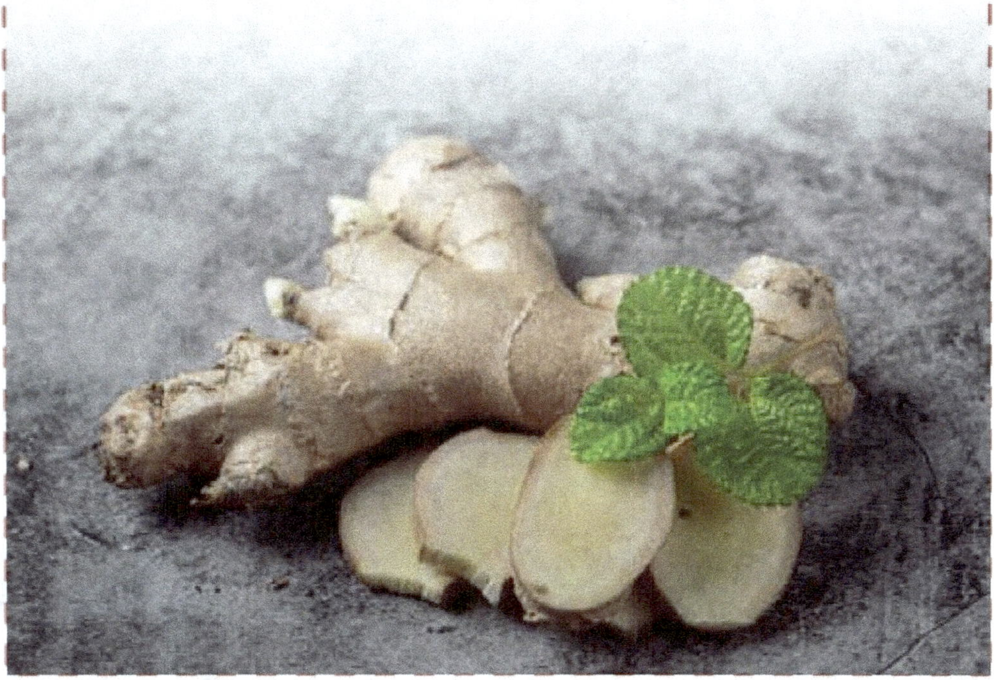

Food to *Fight Cancer*

Specific steps that you can take to fight cancer

Ellagic acid, available in foods such as pomegranate, pecans and berries, causes the cancer cells to go through the normal apoptosis process (programmed cell death) without damaging healthy cells. Ellagic acid stimulates the mitochondria to induce this process of apoptosis (typically called mitochondrial pathway of apoptosis). This action is associated with mitochondrial electrical activation in a process called depolarization.

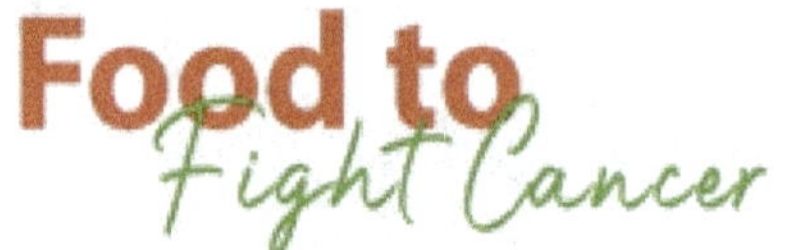

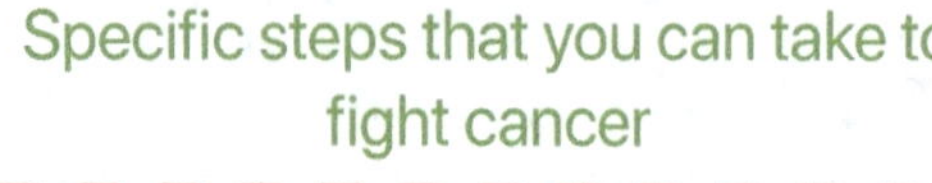

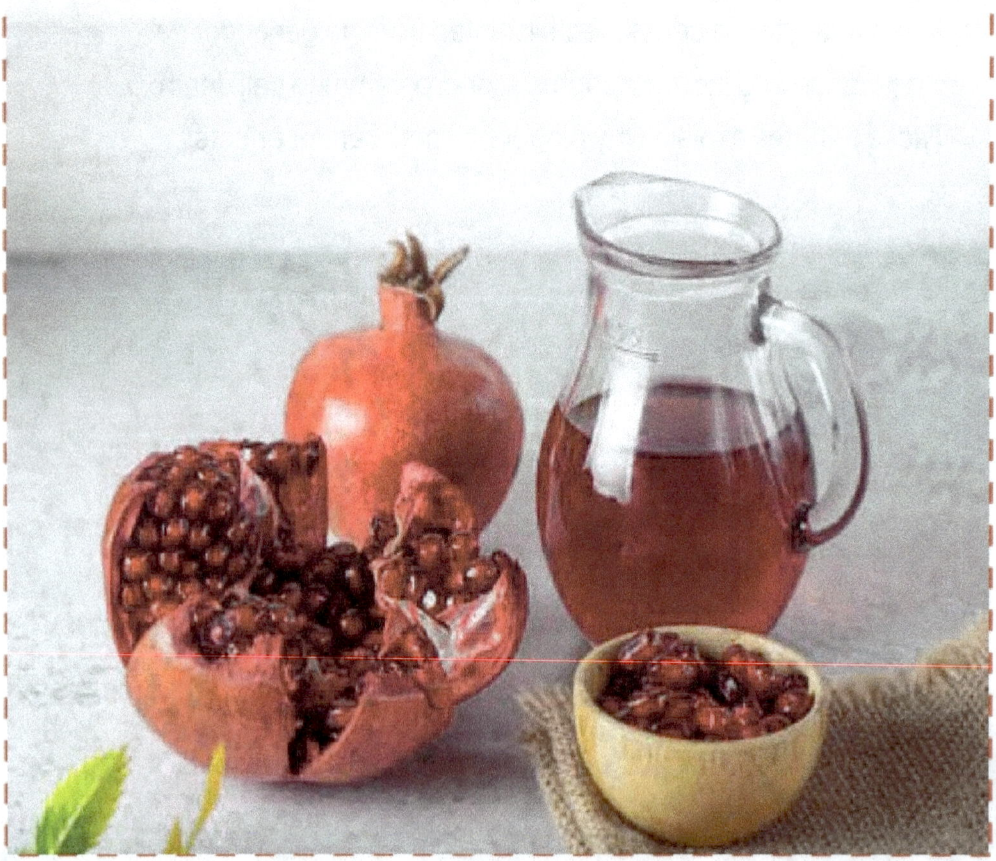

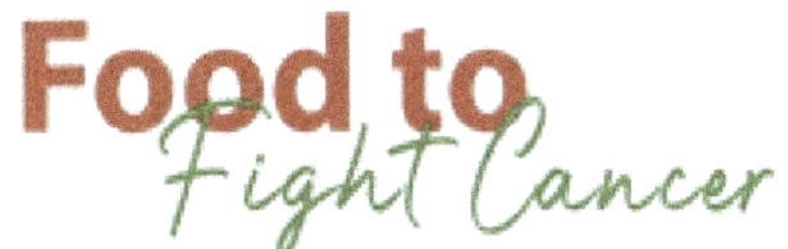

Quercetin may induce apoptosis by direct activation of mitochondrial pathways that lead to programmed cell death in **cancer** cells.

Additionally, it affects the signal interaction between cells in a way that also induces apoptosis.

Fruits and vegetables - particularly citrus fruits, apples, onions, parsley, sage and tea - are the primary dietary sources of quercetin.

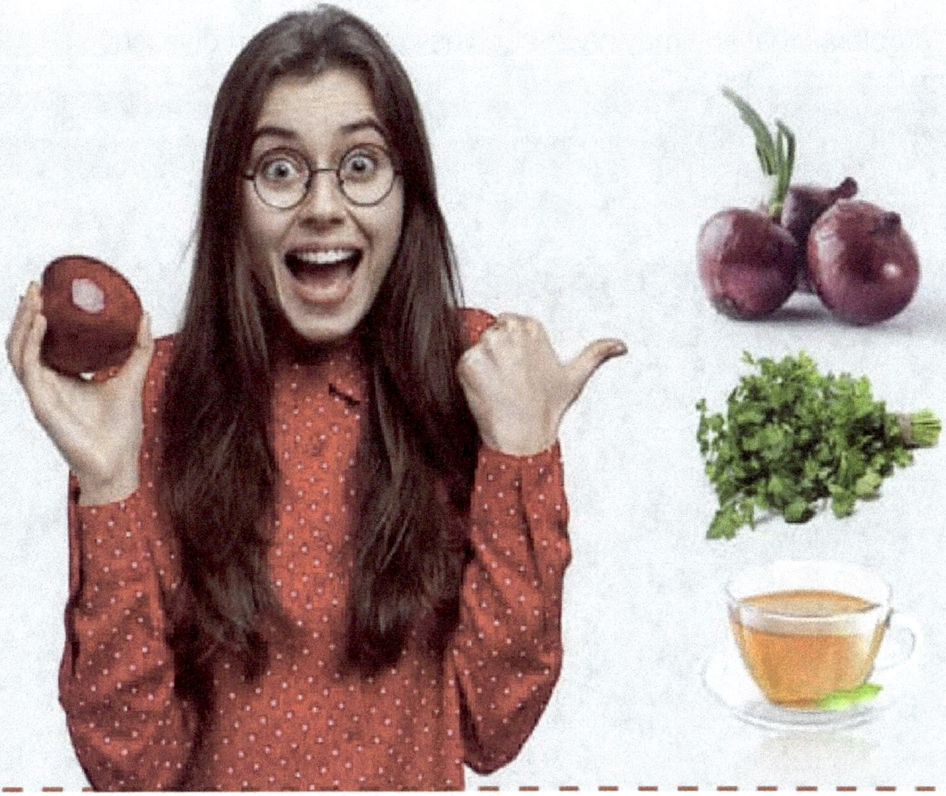

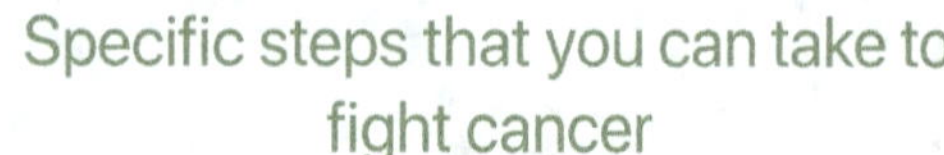

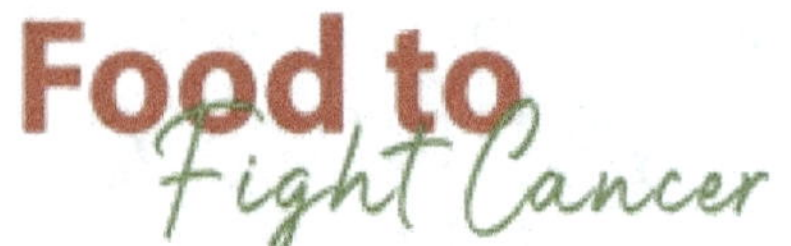

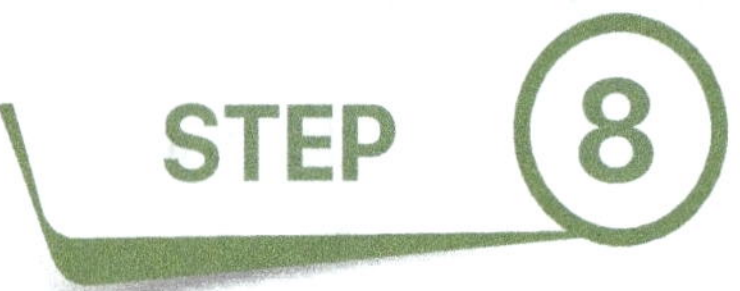

Boost your immune system

Holding your breath underwater for a period of time (apnea) can lower blood oxygen levels in the body and lead to contraction of the spleen.

This splenic contraction pushes millions of immune cells (white blood cells) into our blood and may thus – at least in theory - assist in fighting **cancer** cells.

You should consult your personal doctor before using such an approach to make sure that it does not aggravate other health problems that you may have, such as coronary heart disease.

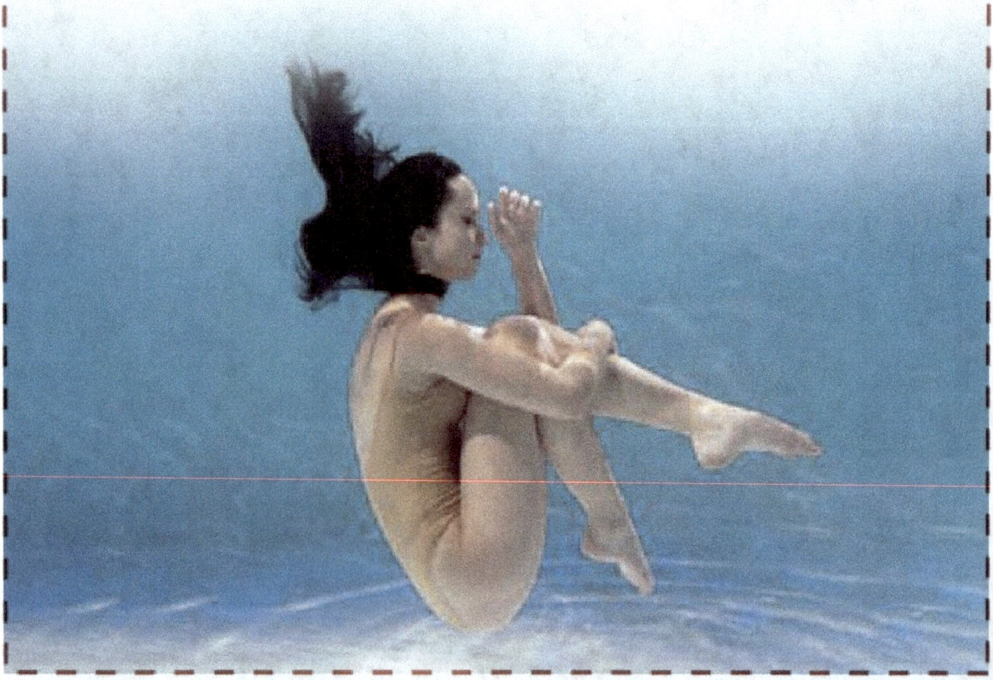

Food to Fight Cancer

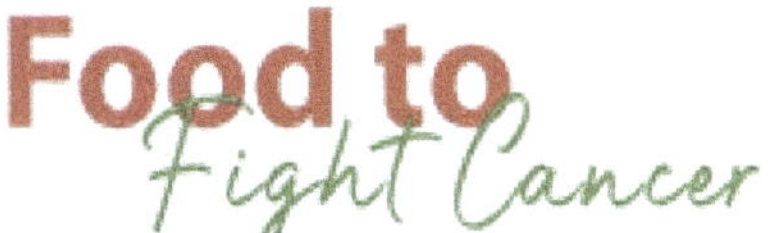

One likely way by which exercise exerts its effect on cancer is by altering the function of the immune system.

Cells of the innate immune system (i.e., macrophage, natural killer cells and neutrophils) are first-line defenders against **cancer**.

Moderate exercise may have an anti-**cancer** effect as it increases the activity of these cells in the body.

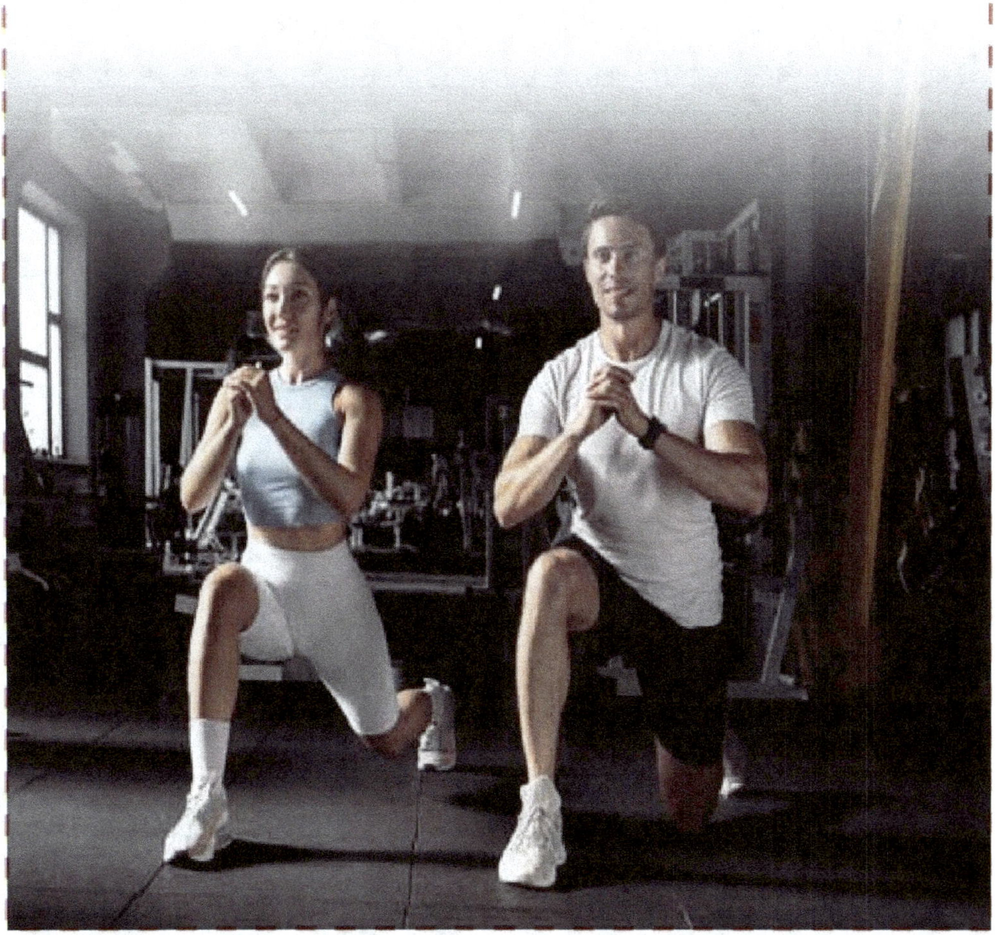

Food to *Fight Cancer*

Specific steps that you can take to fight cancer

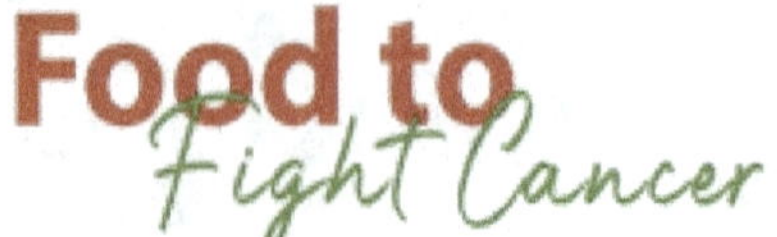

Research has shown that high temperatures can damage and kill **cancer** cells, usually with minimal injury to normal tissues.

By killing **cancer** cells and damaging proteins and structures within cells, hyperthermia may actually shrink tumors.

Cold exposure after heat may cause mobilization of circulating white cells and increase immune cell activity.

Swimming in cold water after exposure to high temperature (e.g., in a sauna) may thus be a useful adjunct in fighting **cancer**.

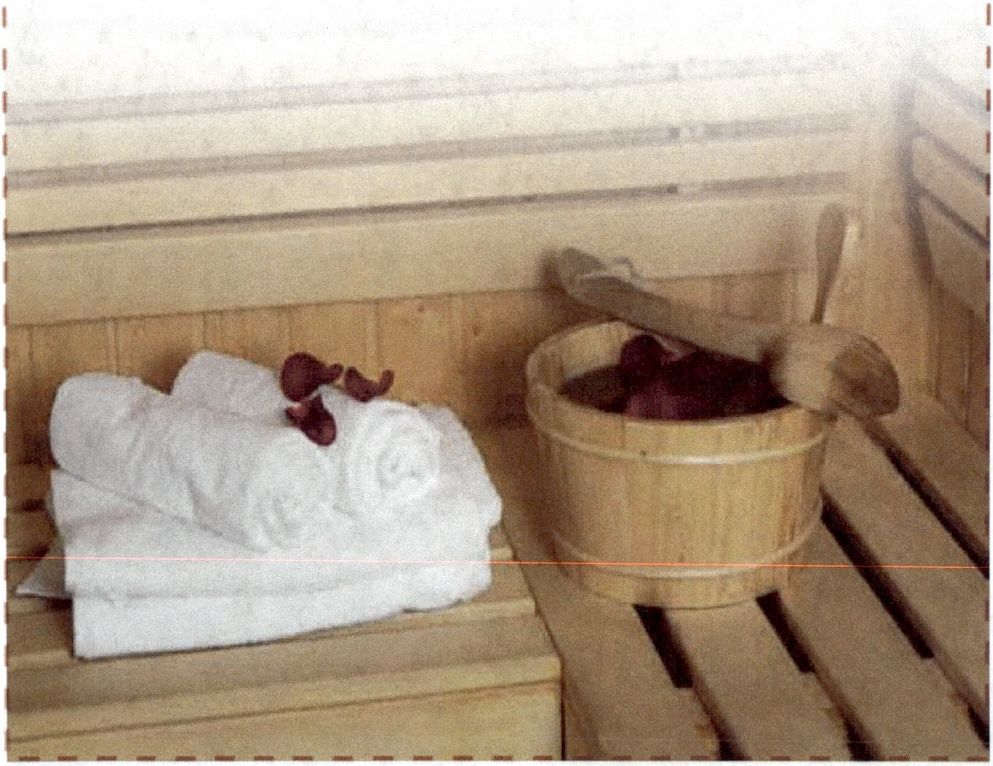

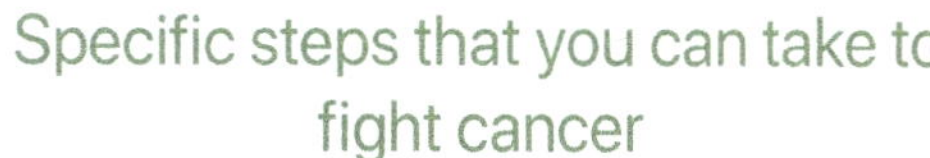

Food to Fight Cancer

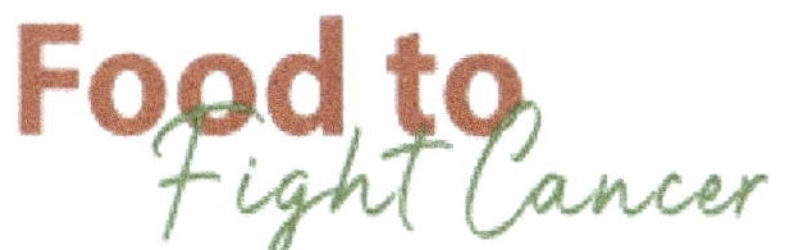

STEP 9

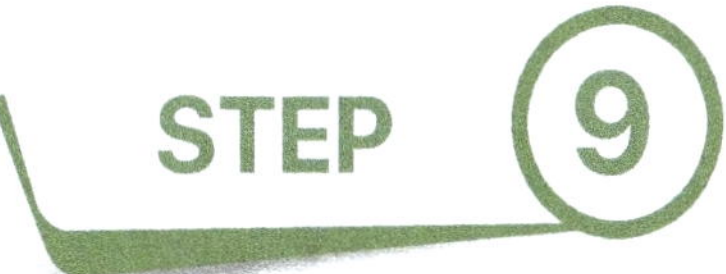

Inhibit new vessel formation in cancer cells

Normally cartilage is located in areas where movement is needed. In normal circumstances, cartilage does not have blood vessels as this would cause bleeding during movement.

The lack of blood vessels in cartilage is due to the presence of a biological compound that inhibits blood vessel formation (angiogenesis).

This factor - the anti-angiogenesis factor - is the secret behind the lack of blood vessels in cartilage.

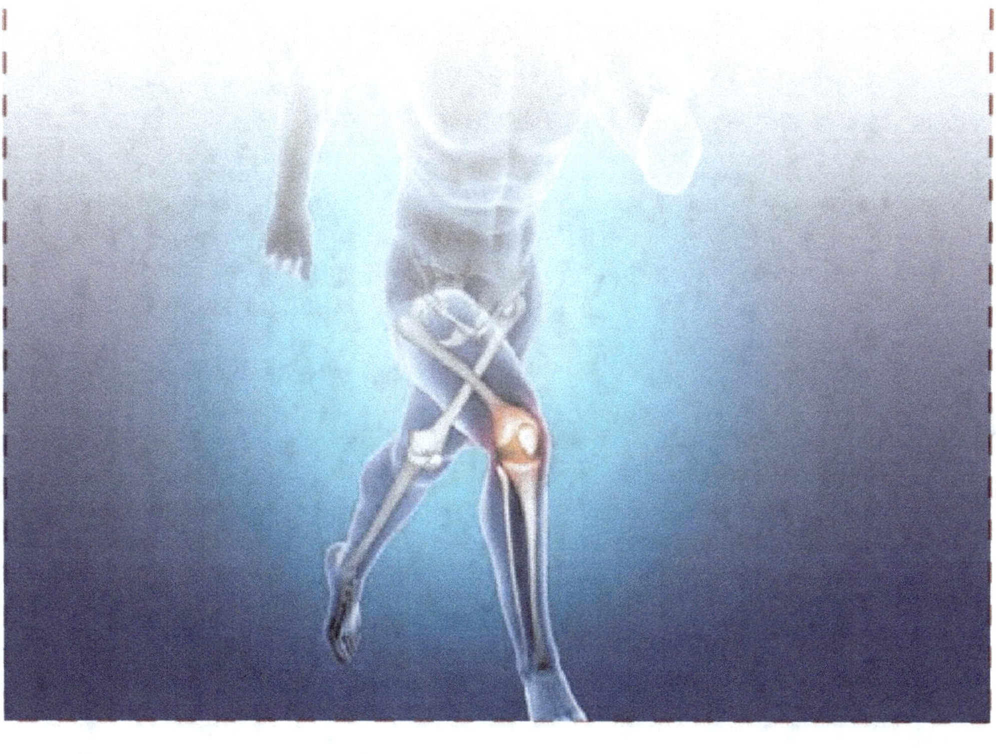

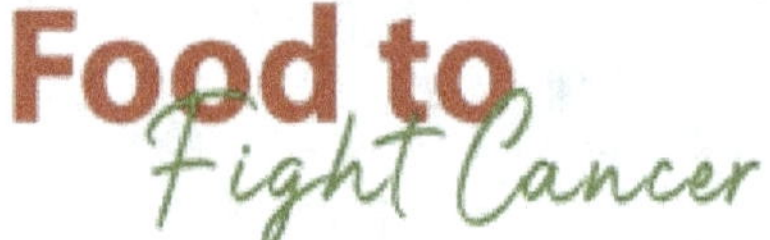

Food to *Fight Cancer*

Specific steps that you can take to fight cancer

Research has shown that high temperatures can damage and kill **cancer** cells, usually with minimal injury to normal tissues.

By killing **cancer** cells and damaging proteins and structures within cells, hyperthermia may actually shrink tumors.

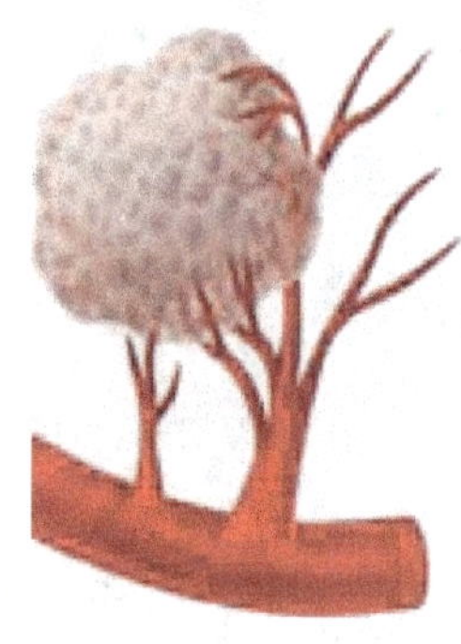

Cold exposure after heat may cause mobilization of circulating white cells and increase immune cell activity.

Swimming in cold water after exposure to high temperature (e.g., in a sauna) may thus be a useful adjunct in fighting **cancer**.

This concept led to the use of shark cartilage in the form of a supplement to provide anti-angiogenesis factors in an attempt to defeat **cancer**.

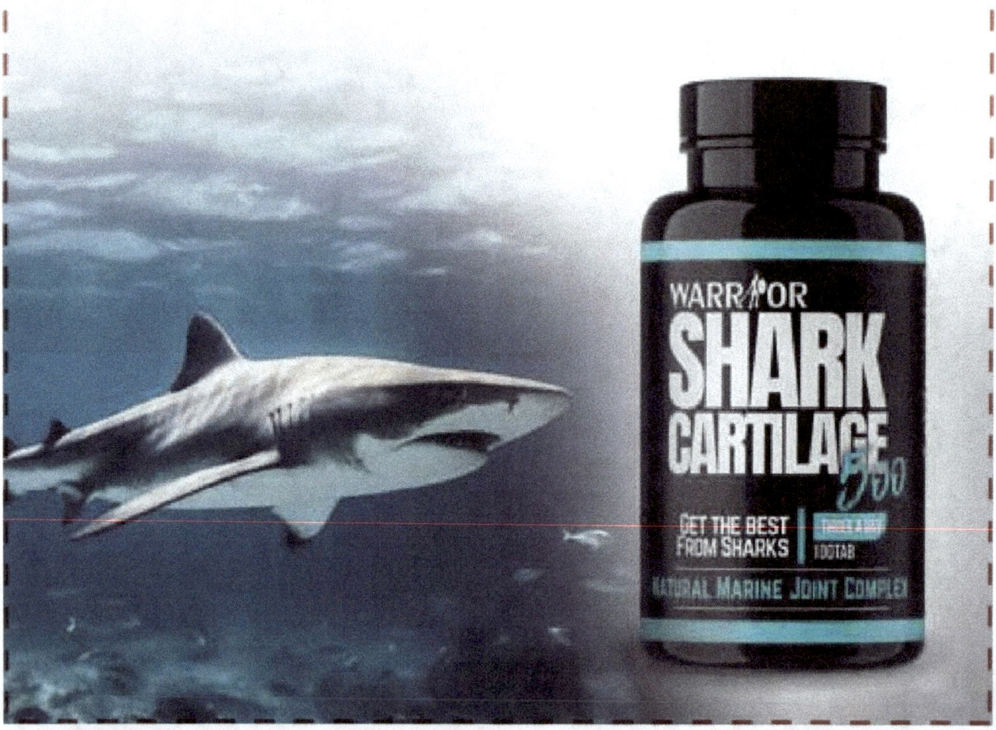

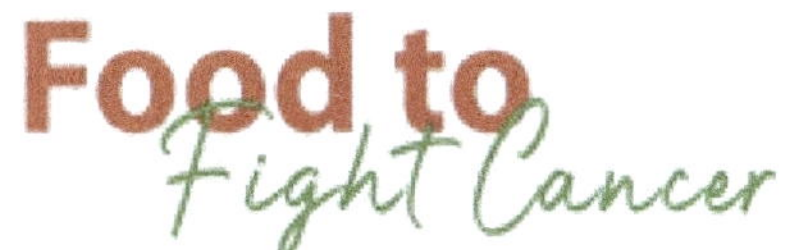

Food to Fight Cancer

Other food components that can inhibit angiogenesis new blood formation in **cancer** cells include:

01 Curcumin

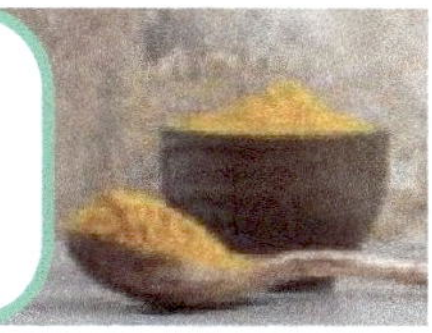

02 Grape seed extract

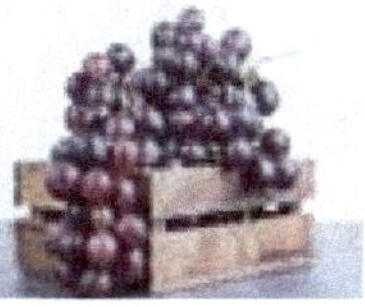

03 Ginkgo biloba

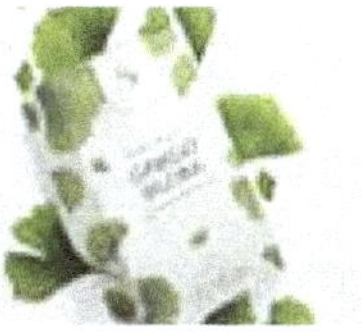

04 Quercetin

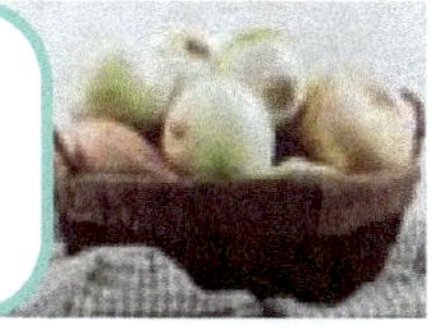

05 Ginger

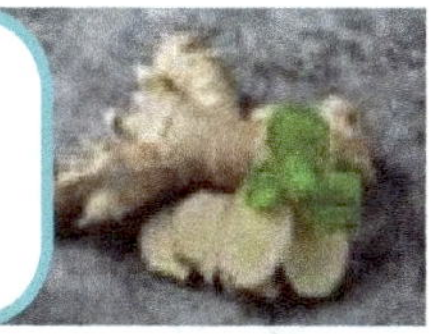

These herbs may exert their anti-angiogenesis effects through affecting gene expression, signal processing and enzyme activities.

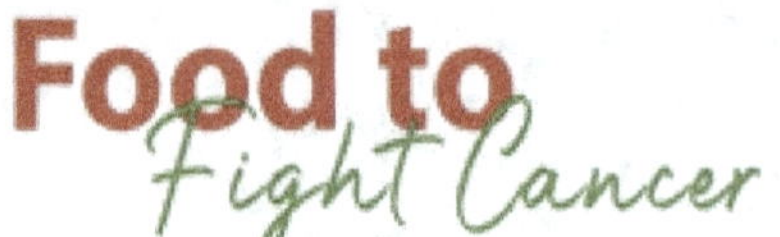

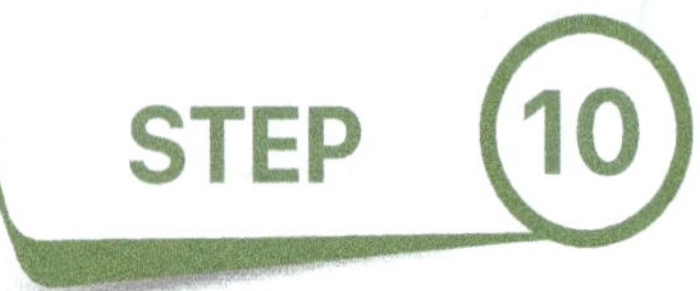

Inhibit degrading enzymes of cancer cells (proteases)

The main difference between a benign and malignant tumor is the ability of the malignant cells to invade normal tissue and spread or metastasize to distant sites throughout the body.

It is the ability to form metastasis which makes **cancer** such a difficult disease to treat.

The most likely mechanism by which **cancer** invades adjacent tissues is via secreting protein-degrading enzymes called proteases.

These proteases mediate metastasis by catalyzing degradation of the extracellular matrix and basement membranes.

Inhibition of these enzymes could open up new therapeutic approaches for the control of malignancy.

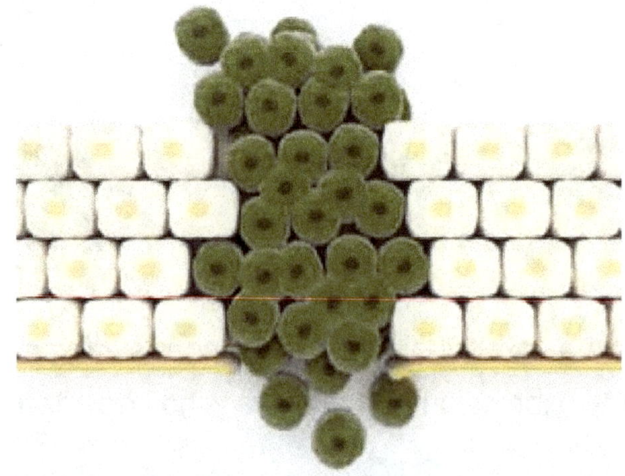

Food to *Fight Cancer*

Specific steps that you can take to fight cancer

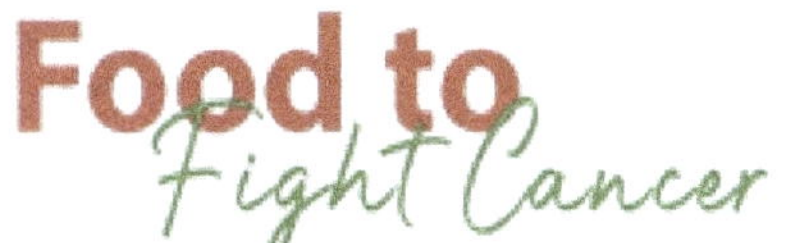

Sulforaphane, a dietary component of broccoli/broccoli sprouts, inhibits the proteases that allow **cancer** to degrade the extracellular matrix around it.

Broccoli sprouts have the highest vegetable concentration of sulforaphane.

Sulforaphane is also found in Brussels sprouts, cauliflower, Chinese broccoli, mustard, daikon, turnip, radish, capers and watercress.

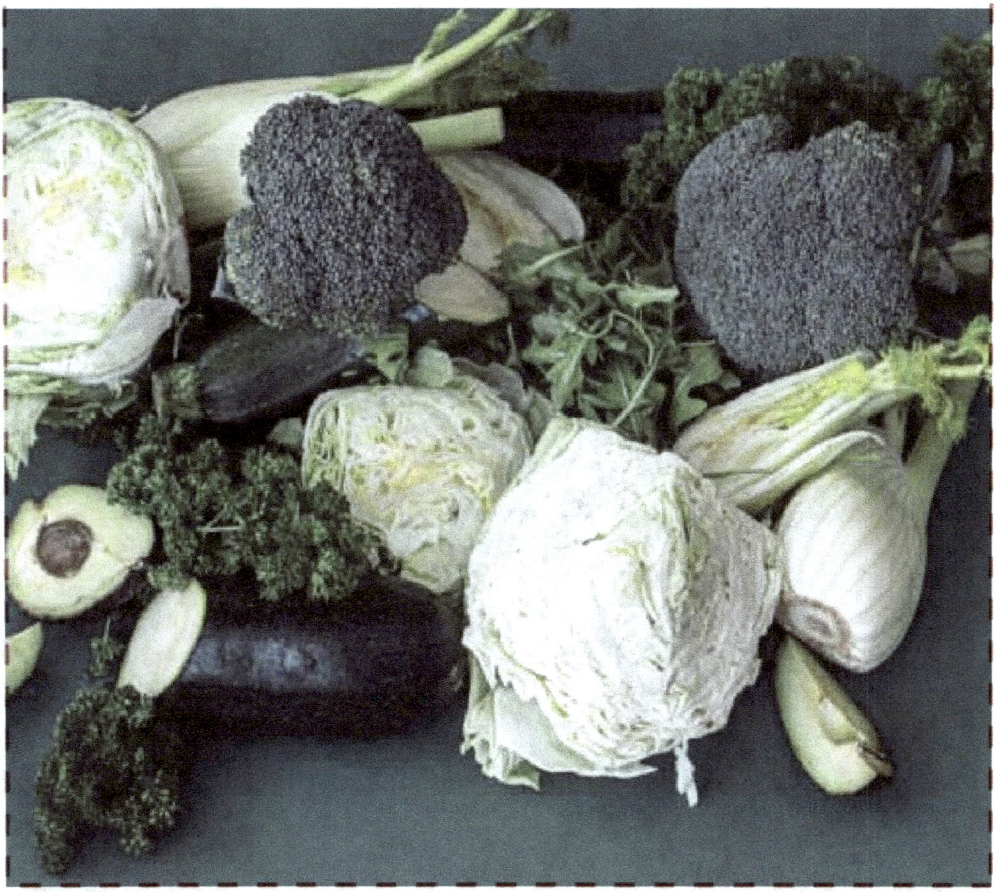

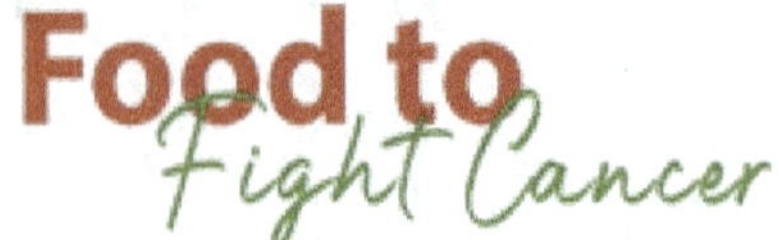

Sulforaphane doesn't exist independently in plants; it must be created through a specific enzymatic process.

The enzyme required is myrosinase.

Myrosinase transforms the compound glucoraphanin (the inert form of suforaphane) into sulforaphane upon damage to the plant.

So, now you know why you need to properly chew the plant before swallowing - no chewing, no sulforaphane.

**No chewing,
no sulforaphane.**

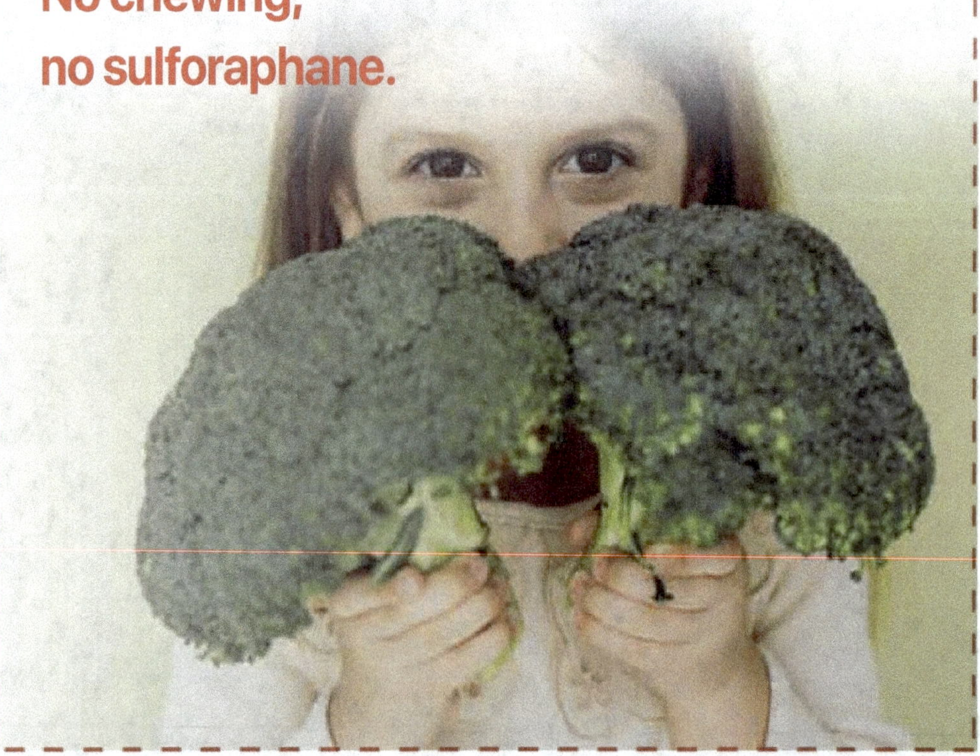

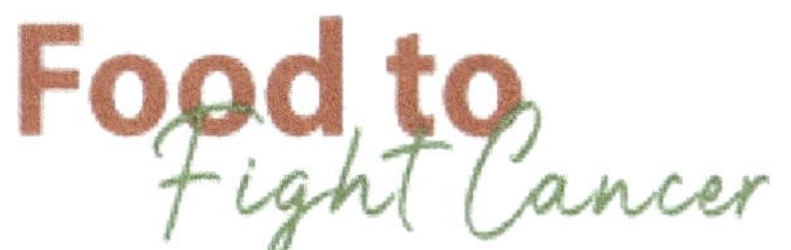

Food to Fight Cancer

STEP 11

Increase your intake of superfoods

Garlic contains an abundance of chemical compounds that have been shown to possess beneficial anti-**cancer** effects.

Such effects appear to be related to the presence of organosulfur compounds (OSC), predominantly allyl derivatives, which have been shown to inhibit carcinogenesis.

Organosulfur compounds modulate the activity of several enzymes that activate (cytochrome P450s) or detoxify carcinogens.

Additionally, these compounds inhibit the formation of DNA adducts in several target tissues.

Garlic also induces apoptosis of **cancer** cells.

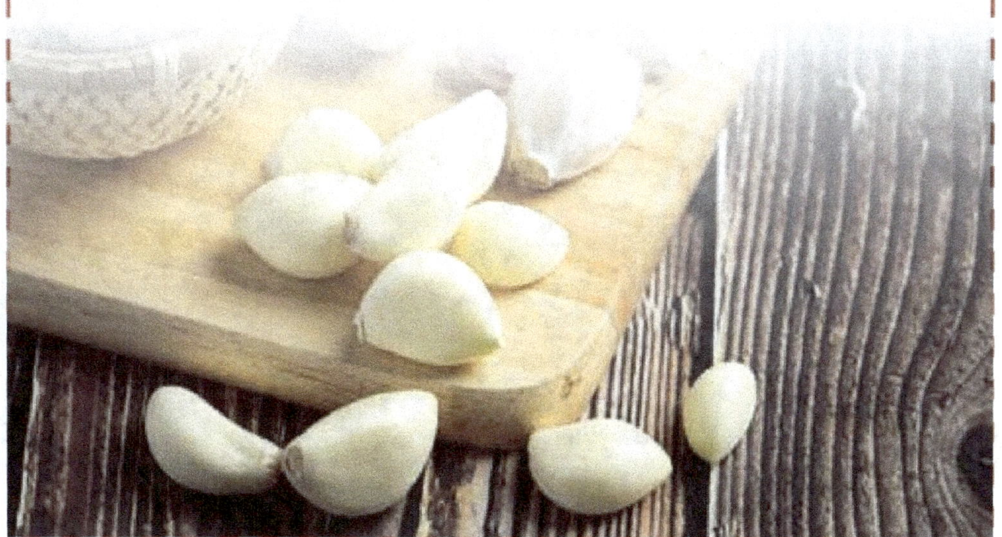

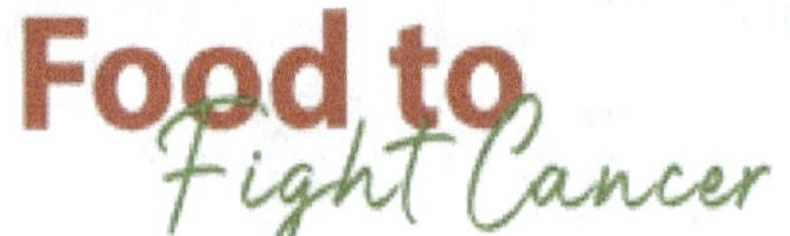

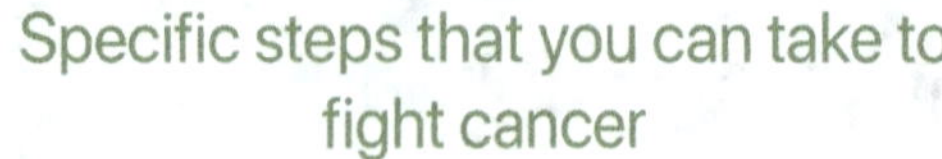

Legumes, which include beans, lentils and peas, along with many other varieties, also have the ability to fight **cancer**.

One of the active ingredients in beans that scientists believe may play a role in **cancer** prevention is saponins, a protease inhibitor.

Saponins in legumes have shown the ability to inhibit the spread of **cancer** cells.

They do this by inhibiting the **cancer** proteases that destroy nearby cells, which in turn prevents the **cancer** from being able to metastasize.

In this context, it is also important to mention that phytic acid in legumes has shown the ability to significantly slow the progression of tumors.

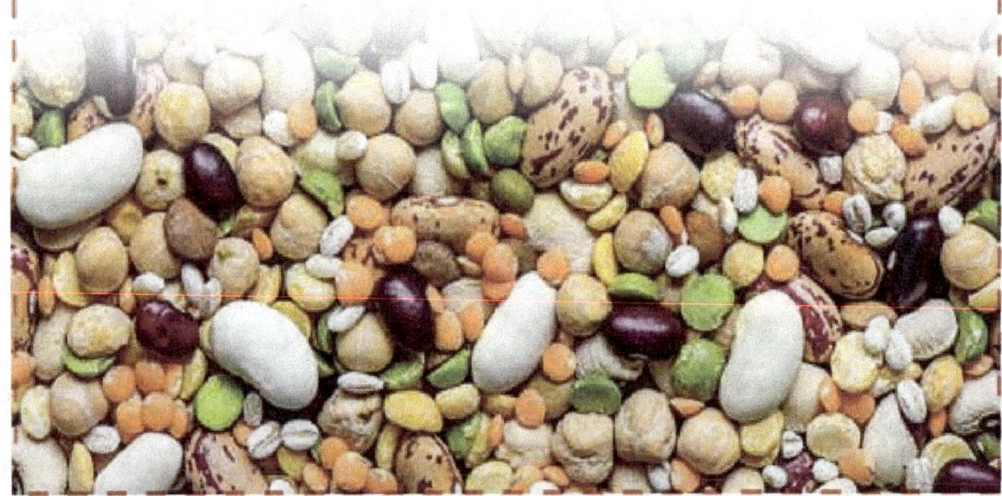

Food to *Fight Cancer*

Specific steps that you can take to fight cancer

Honey is a natural product that shows potential effects to inhibit or suppress the development and progression of tumors and **cancer**. Its anti-**cancer** effects are mediated via diverse mechanisms, including cell cycle arrest, induction of cell death (apoptosis), modulation of oxidative stress, amelioration of inflammation, modulation of growth factors signaling, and inhibition of angiogenesis in **cancer** cells.

Honey is highly and selectively cytotoxic against tumors and **cancer** cells while it is non-cytotoxic to normal cells.

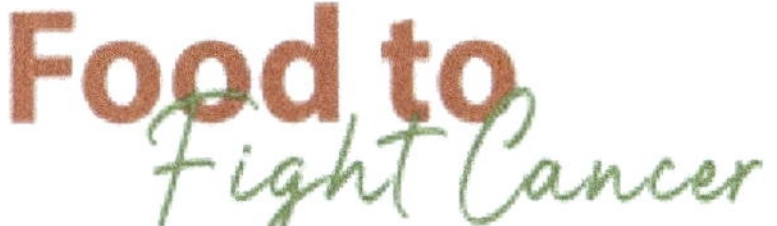

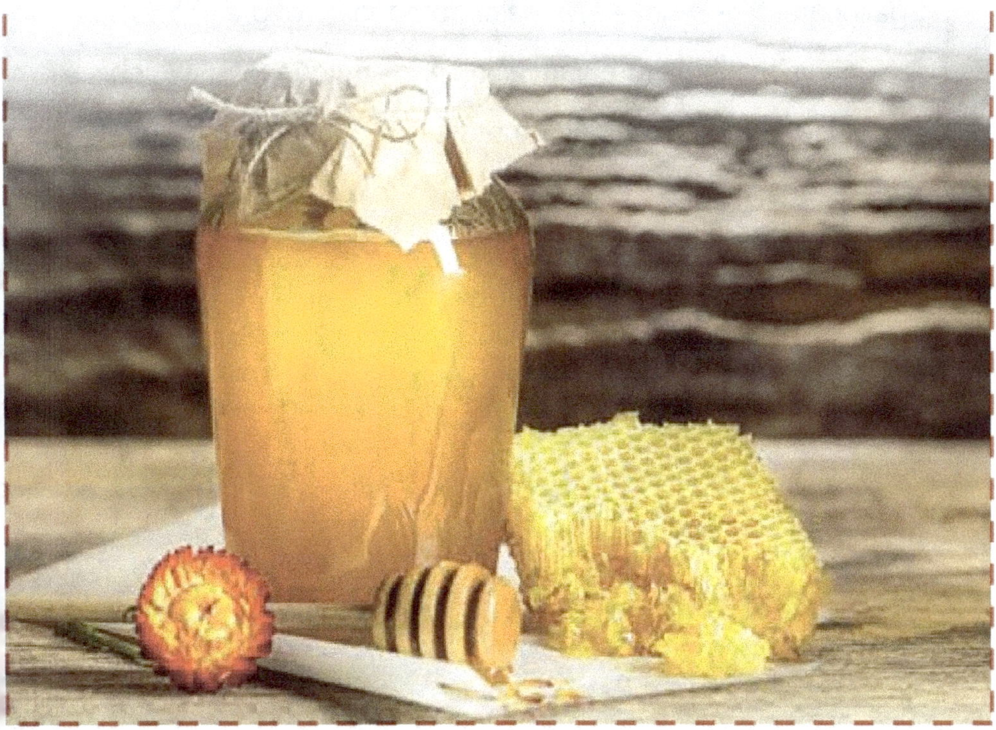

Food to Fight Cancer

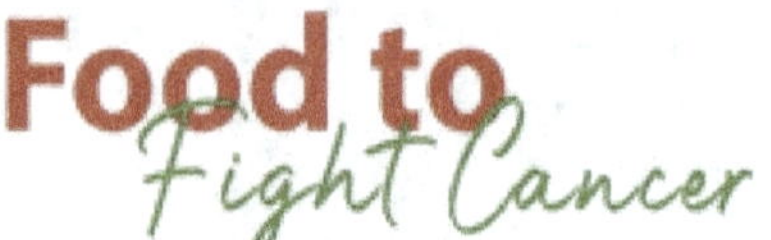

Metastasis is the main factor accounting for the majority of **cancer** deaths.

As such, therapeutic strategies to prevent the development of metastases have the potential to greatly reduce **cancer** mortality rates.

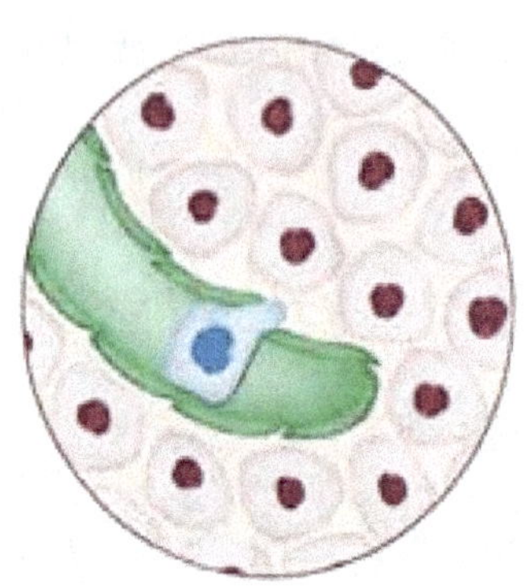

The possible **cancer**-preventive attributes of green tea constituents has been studied extensively.

The amount of experimental evidence documenting the properties of green tea, which affects multiple signaling pathways against metastasis of **cancer**, is increasing rapidly.

Epigallocatechin-3-gallate, a major component of green tea, has been shown to inhibit tumor invasion and angiogenesis, which are essential for tumor growth and metastasis.

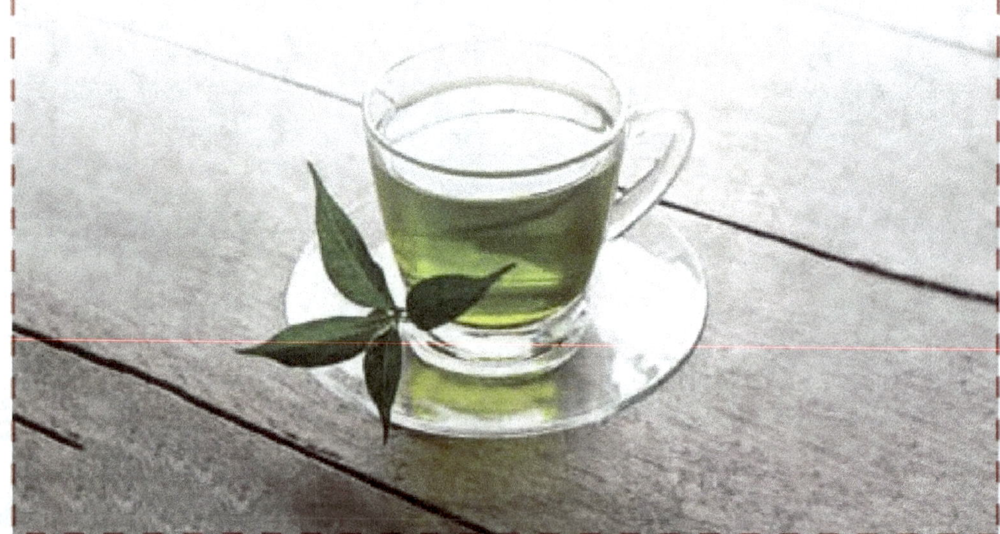

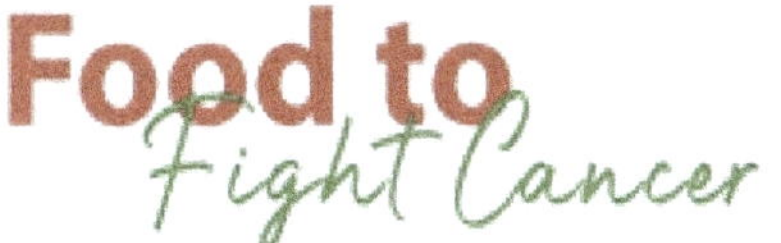

Food to Fight Cancer

Extra virgin olive oil, a central component of the Mediterranean diet, contains an abundance of phenolic antioxidants that are potent inhibitors of reactive oxygen species and is associated with a reduced risk of several types of human **cancer**.

Oleocanthal, a phenolic compound in extra virgin olive oil, has the ability to kill **cancer** cells.

In some tests, oleocanthal induced cell death in all **cancer** cells examined in as little as thirty minutes.

Oleocanthal caused **cancer** cell death by affecting the lysosomes (these are vesicles where **cancer** cells store their enzymes).

This amazing effect of olive oil on **cancer** cells is mediated via inhibiting acid sphingomyelinase (ASM) activity, which destabilizes the interaction between proteins necessary for lysosomal membrane stability in the malignant cells.

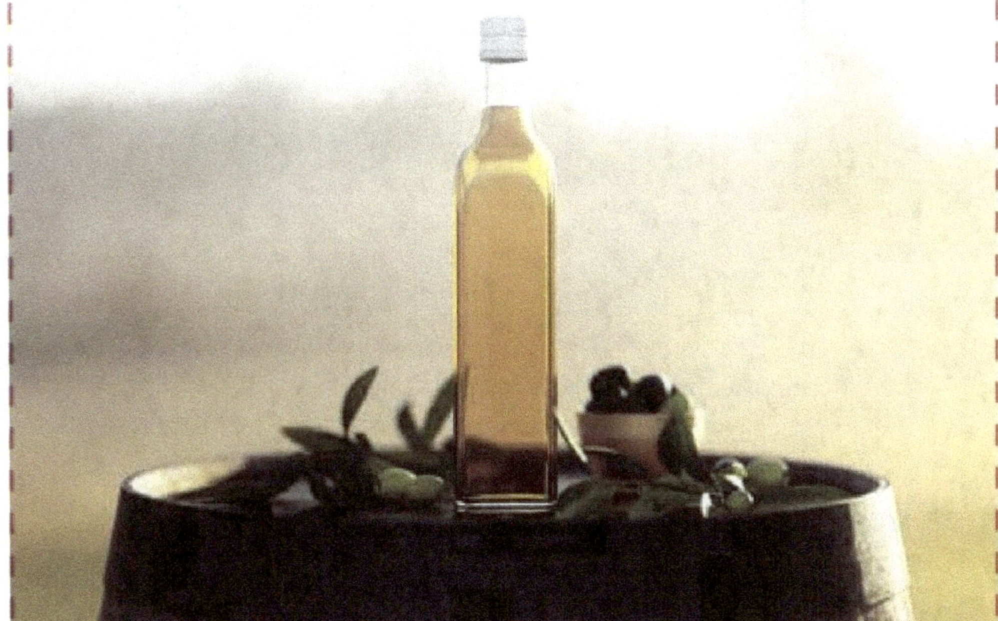

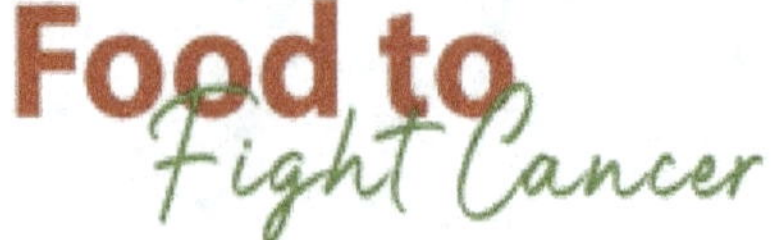

Food to Fight Cancer

Recently, a number of bioactive molecules, including anti-tumor agents, have been identified from various mushrooms.

These include polysaccharides, proteins, fats, glycosides, alkaloids, volatile oils, tocopherols, phenolics, flavonoids, carotenoids, folates, ascorbic acid enzymes, and organic acids.

The polysaccharide, β-glucan, for example, is the most versatile anti-**cancer** compound in mushrooms due to its broad spectrum biological activity.

Their mechanisms of action involve their being recognized as non-self molecules, so they stimulate the immune system to kill **cancer** cells.

Additionally, hispolon, an active polyphenol compound in mushrooms, is also known to possess potent anti-neoplastic properties.

Furthermore, the anti-**cancer** compounds in mushrooms may play a crucial role in suppressing angiogenesis, inducing apoptosis, and eventually inhibiting **cancer** proliferation.

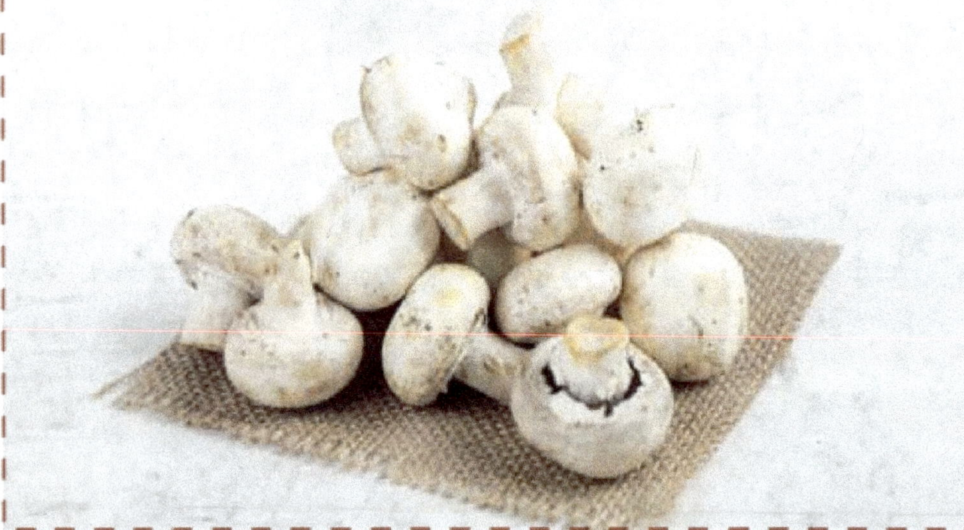

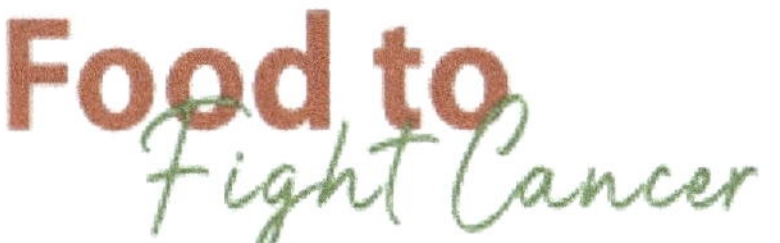

Food to Fight Cancer

Soybean contains a compound called genistein. Genistein inhibits protein tyrosine kinase (PTK), which is involved in the process of activation of **cancer** cells.

Additionally, by blocking several enzymes, it can arrest **cancer** cell growth and proliferation, decrease its ability to spread to and invade adjacent tissues, and inhibit the process of angiogenesis inside malignant cells.

Furthermore, genistein can alter the expression of gangliosides and other carbohydrate antigens to facilitate immune recognition of **cancer** cells which allows our immune system to destroy them.

Soybeans also have high oleic acid content, which could have a potential therapeutic effect in helping to reduce the growth of several types of **cancers**.

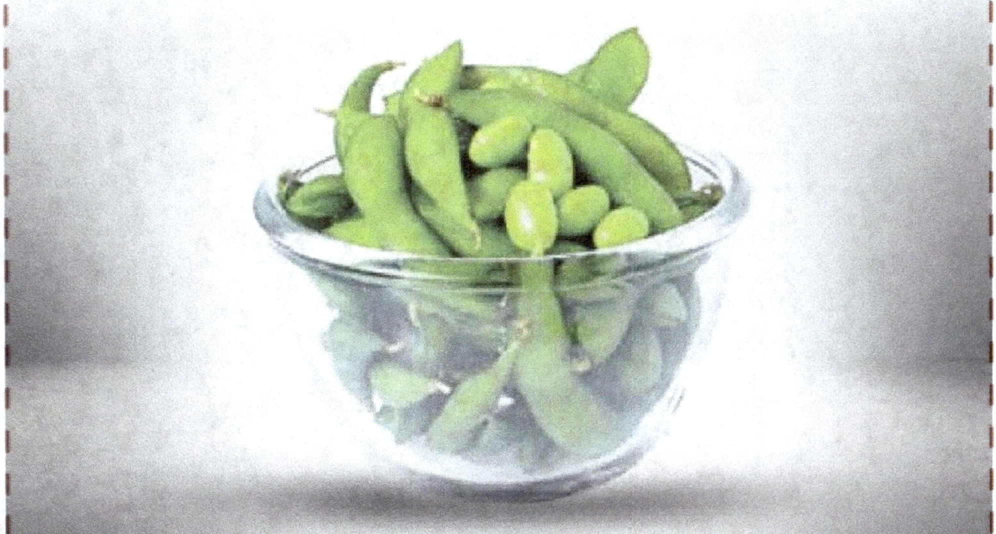

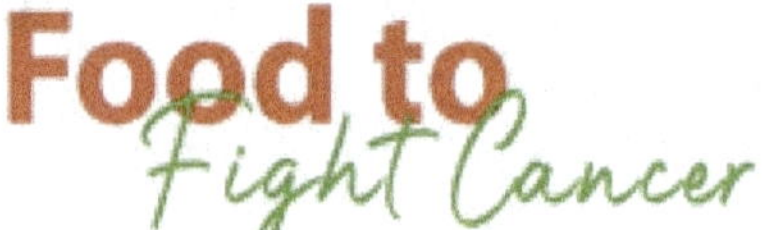

Food to Fight Cancer

Saffron is a spice made from the flower of the saffron plant. The spice is used in cooking as a seasoning for several forms of food, such as rice. It is native to Southwest Asia.

Saffron is considered to be the world's most costly spice, and has been for a long time.

Studies show that saffron is able to suppress - and in some cases reverse - the proliferation of certain human **cancer** cells in culture. Additionally, saffron has been shown to trigger apoptosis (the programmed cell death of **cancer** cells) in a variety of **cancer** cell lines.

In fact, all three major components of saffron - crocin, crocetin, and safranal - have shown powerful apoptosis-inducing properties. Saffron induces programmed cell death in **cancer** cells via activation of P53.

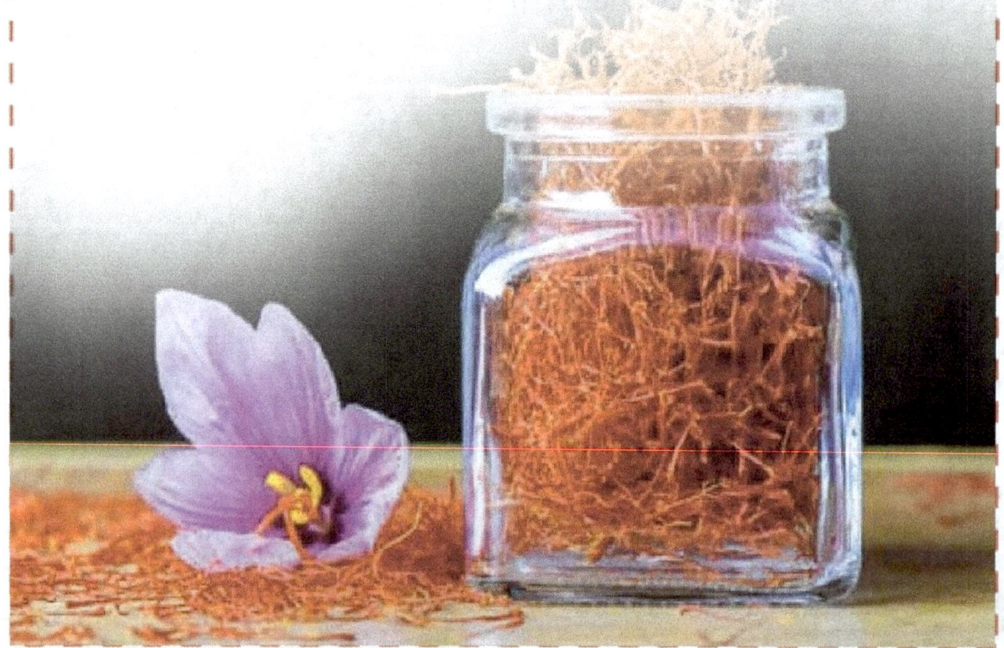

Food to
Fight Cancer

Eggplant - which is a member of the same family as tomatoes and potatoes - contains biological compounds called glycoalkaloids. Several studies have shown that these compounds have anti-**cancer** attributes.

Additionally, the plant contains flavonoids with powerful antioxidant properties. This adds to the anticancer effect of eggplant.

The plant also contains many kinds of alkaloids, such as solanine, cucurbitacin, choline and so on, which have been proven to have an anti-**cancer** ability.

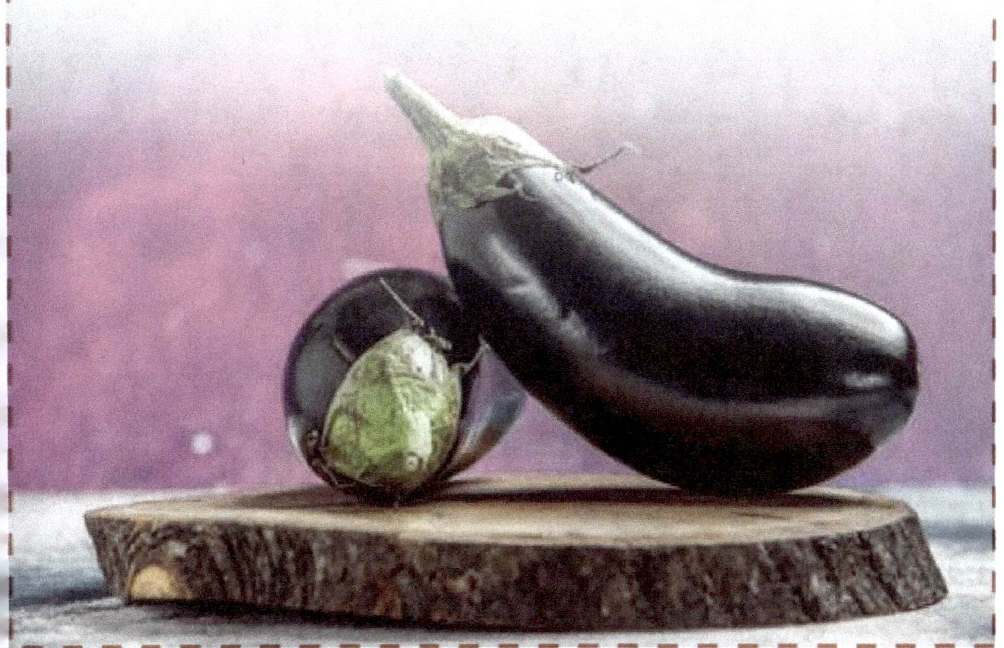

Food to Fight Cancer

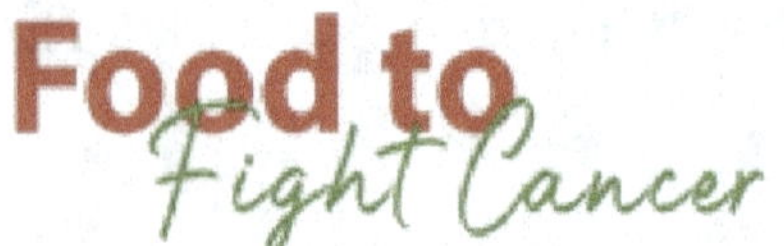

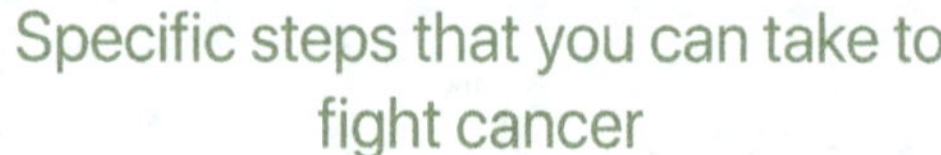

In recent years, many studies have been conducted on the anti-**cancer** effects of **Ferula assa-foetida** (an Indian herb) .

Some compounds isolated from this herb have shown to provide useful pharmacological properties.

These compounds include Ferulic acid and Umbelliferon (a coumarin compound). Both have antitumor effects.

Ferula assa-foetida can be taken as an Indian herb with food, a tincture, and as supplement capsules.

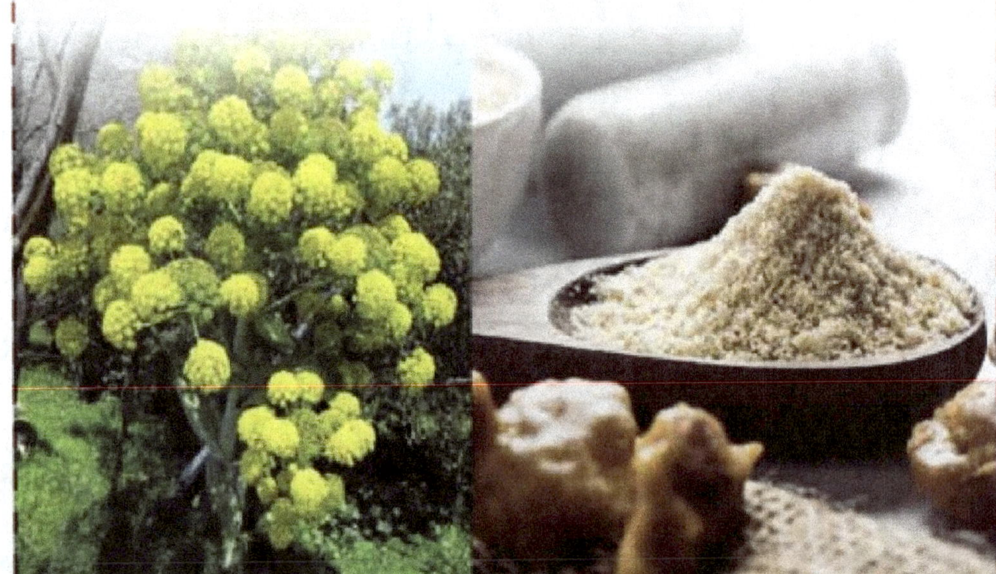

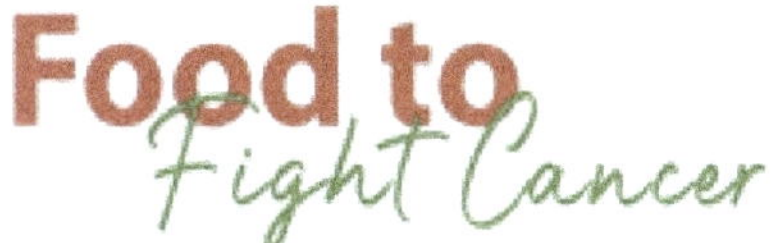

Another promising natural product is **Amygdalin** from **Apricot Kernels** which induces Apoptosis (Programmed cell death of **cancer** cells) and causes Cell Cycle Arrest in the malignant cells.

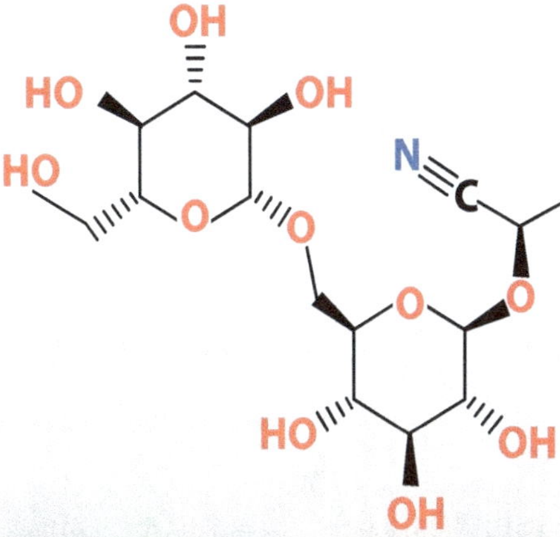

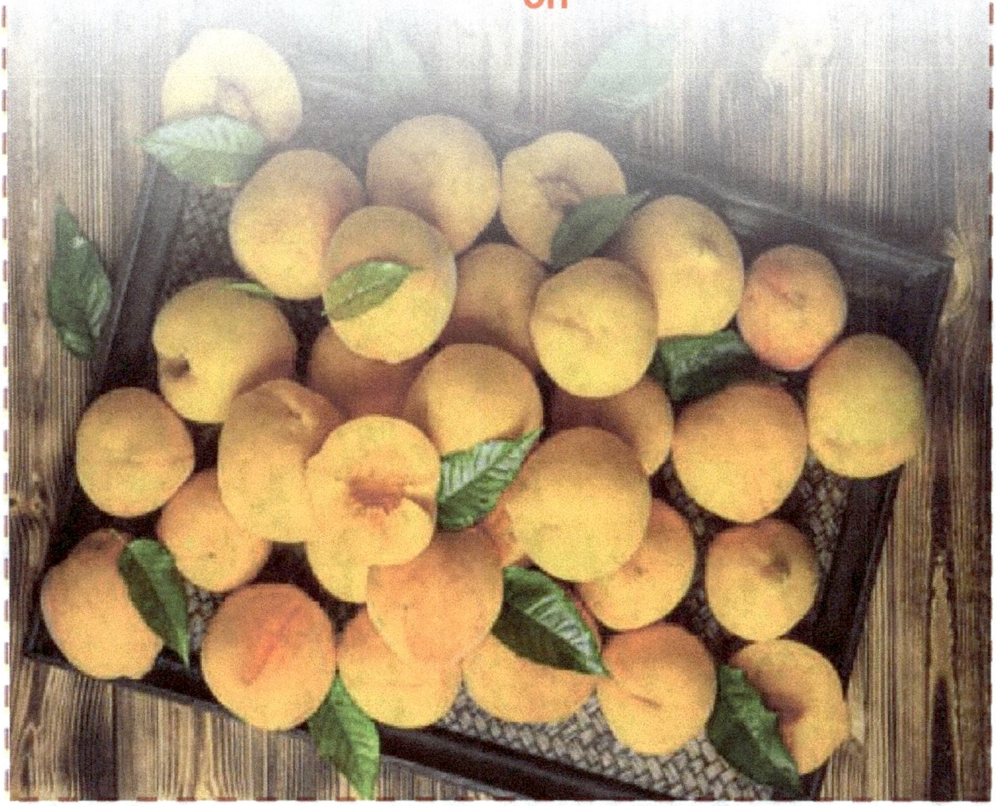

Food to
Fight Cancer

Additionally, **wormwood** (an herb) has shown possible anti-**cancer** properties as documented in multiple preclinical and clinical studies.

Artemisia compounds (ARTs) in wormwood effectively reduce the growth of solid tumors by inhibition of angiogenesis, induction of apoptosis, production of reactive oxygen species and initiation of cell-cycle arrest.

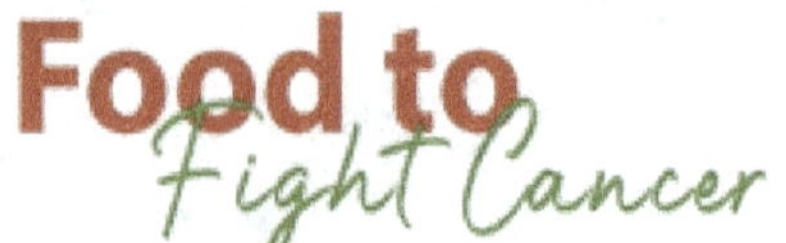

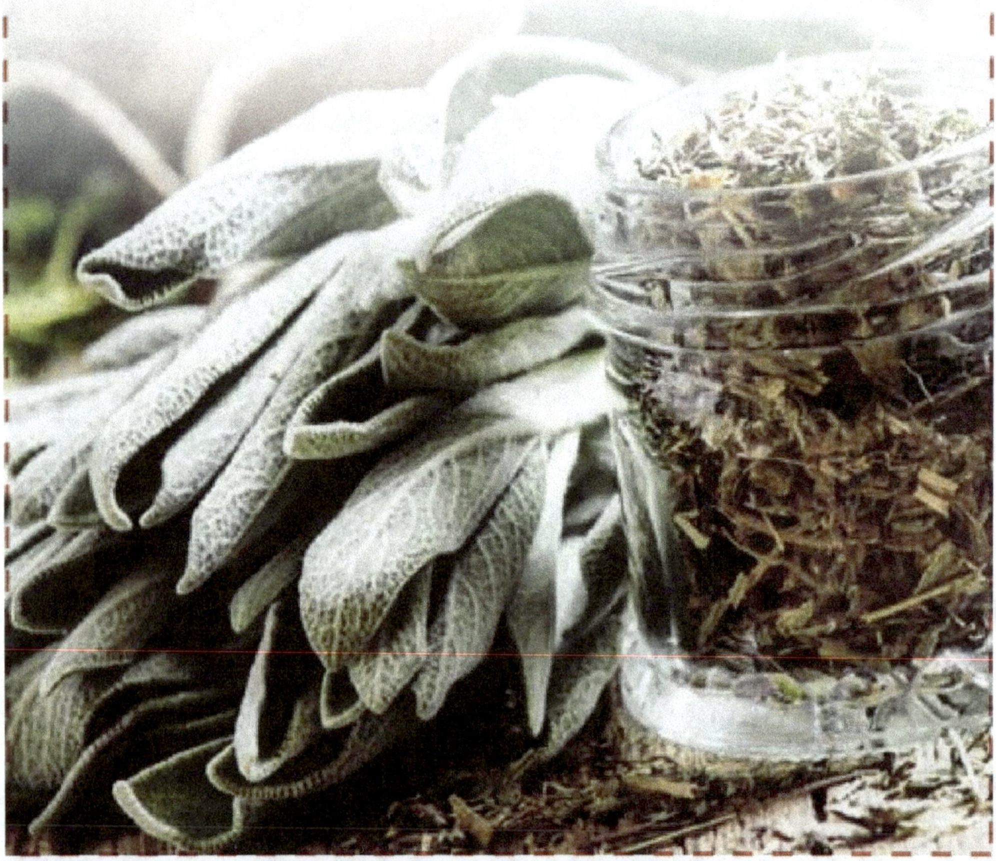

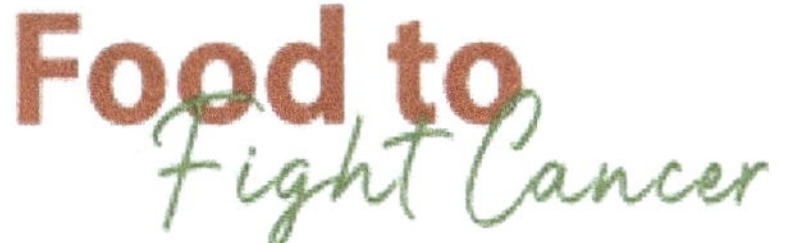

In this context it is also important to mention that citrus peels such as lemon peels contains multiple beneficial anticancer nutrients.

Flavonoids, for example, exist in citrus peels abundantly.

Due to their broad range of pharmacological properties, citrus flavonoids have gained increased attention.

Several studies have indicated that Polymethoxyflavones (PMFs) from citrus peels inhibit **cancer** by mechanisms such as blocking the metastasis cascade, inhibition of **cancer** cell mobility, inducing programmed **cancer** cell death (apoptosis), and by blocking new blood vessel formation in **cancer** calls.

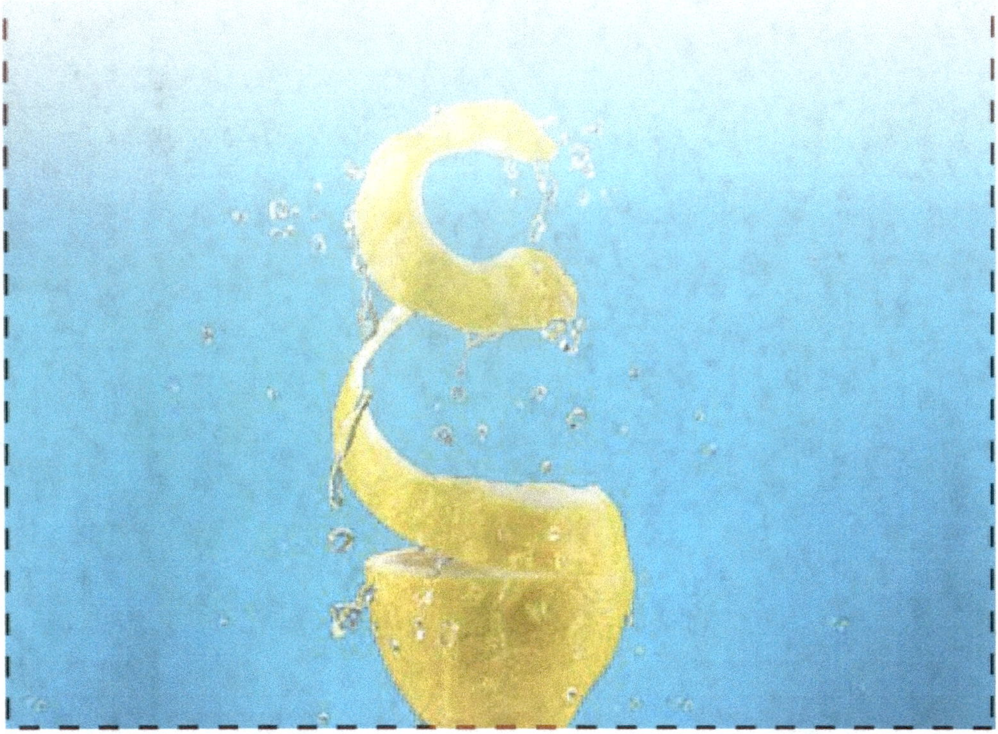

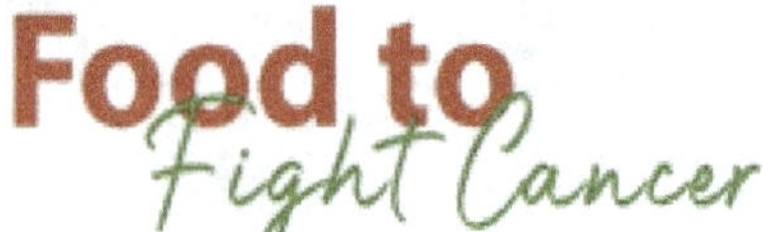

STEP (12)

Decrease contributing factors that may aggravate cancer

As explained earlier, obesity may lead to an increase in insulin and Insulin Like Growth Factor (ILGF) that can aggravate the cancerous process.

Accordingly, decreasing sugar intake to decrease the degree of obesity can be a useful adjunct in the fight against cancer.

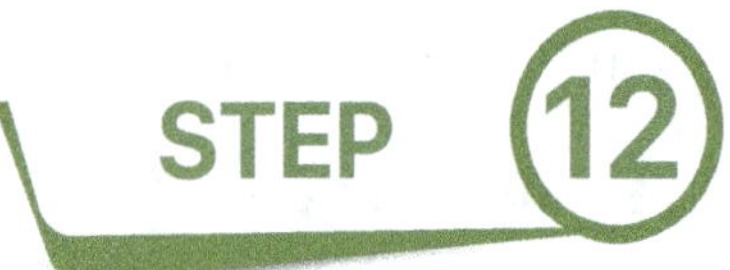

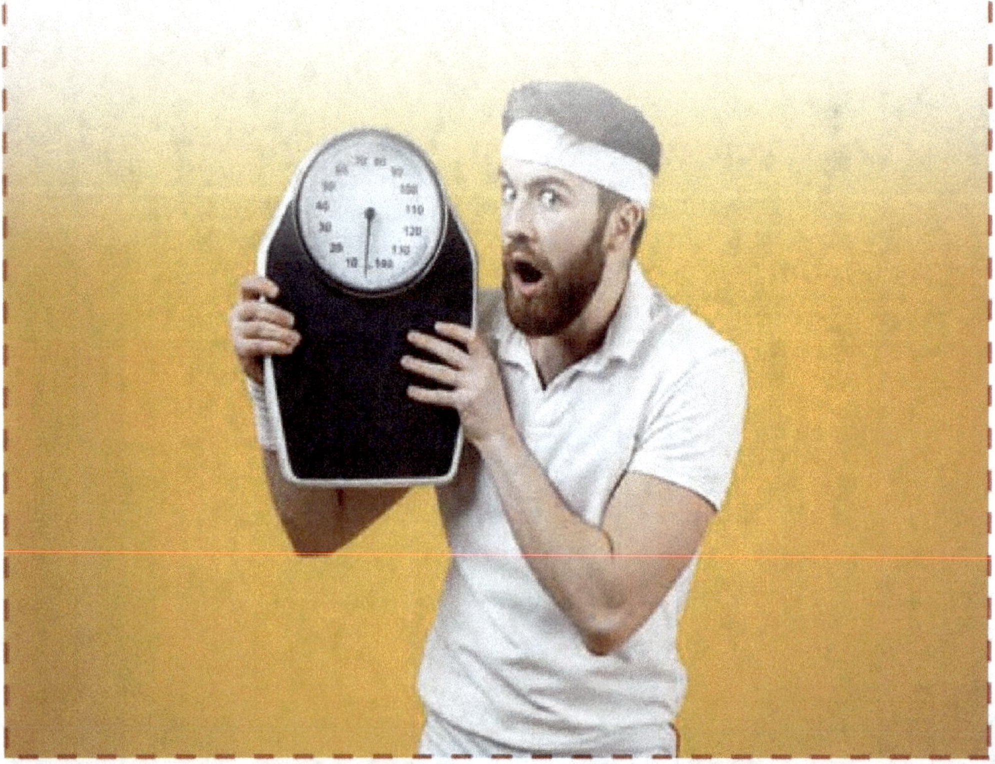

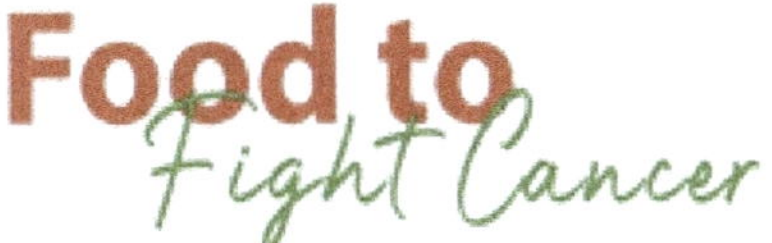

Food to Fight Cancer

Treating any associated psychological depression is important for **cancer** patients.

Some people prefer to use medications to treat their depression. Others use natural methods, such as:

1 - Vitamin D intake, as it can affect brain neurotransmitters in a way to decrease depression

2 - Eating foods that contain serotonin, such as bananas, turkey meat and dark chocolate

3 – Eating foods that contain omega 3 fatty acids, such as fatty fish, walnuts and flaxseed oil

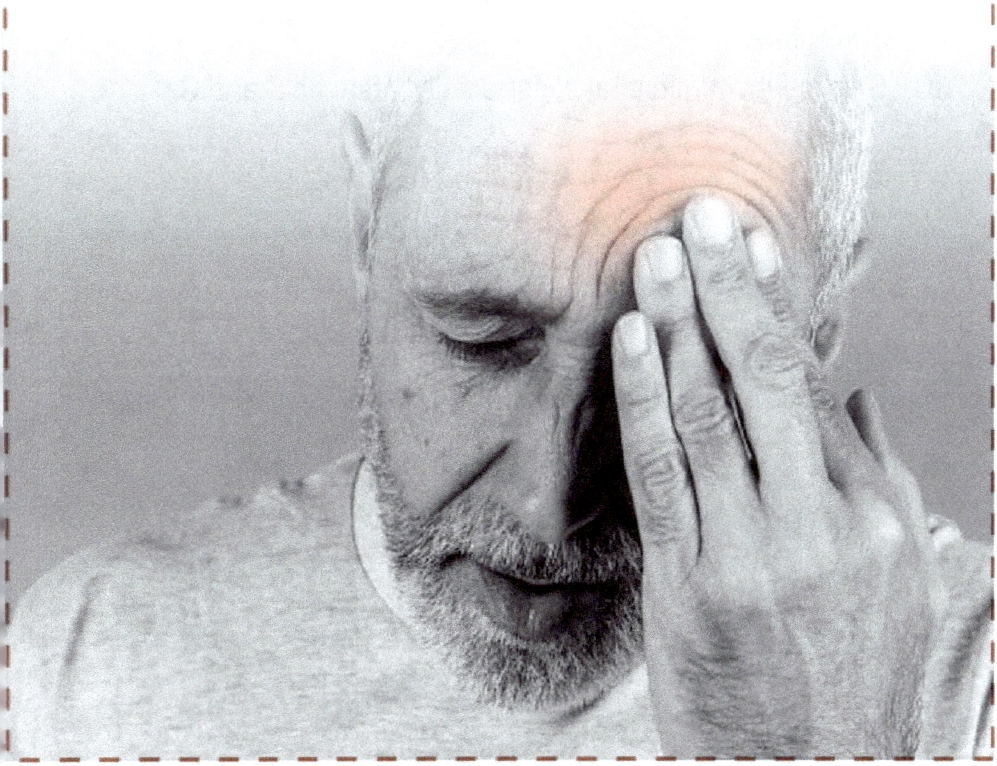

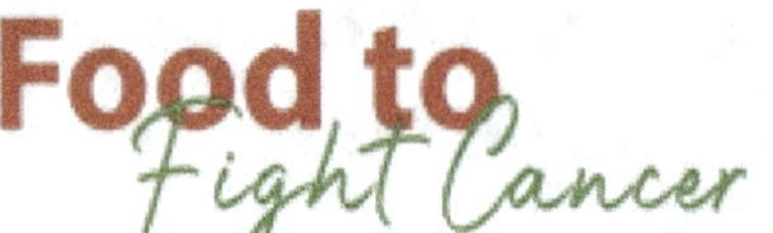

Food to
Fight Cancer

Stress can impede our immune system and thus decrease our ability to fight **cancer**.

Fighting stress must be one of the goals of **cancer** patients.

There are several natural ways to fight stress.

These include:

1 - Decreasing your intake of coffee

2 - Using relaxing herbs, e.g., passionflower

3 - Using essential oils that help you relax

4 - Listening to relaxing music

5 - Relaxing in a spa pool

6 - Exercising

7 - Yoga

8 - Massage

9 - Swimming

10 - Sufficient vitamin intake, especially vitamins B and C

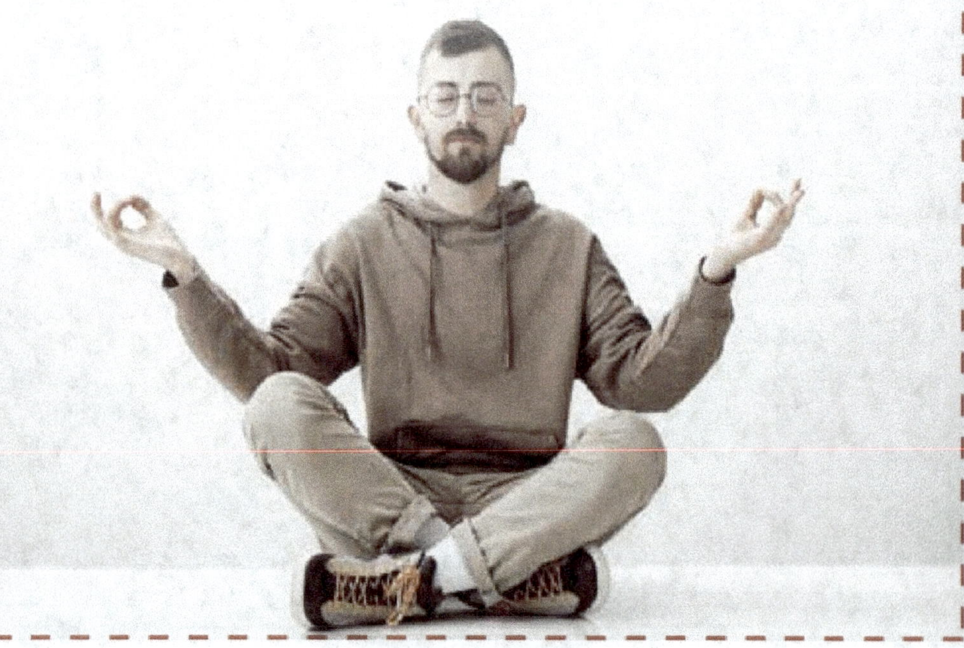

Food to Fight Cancer

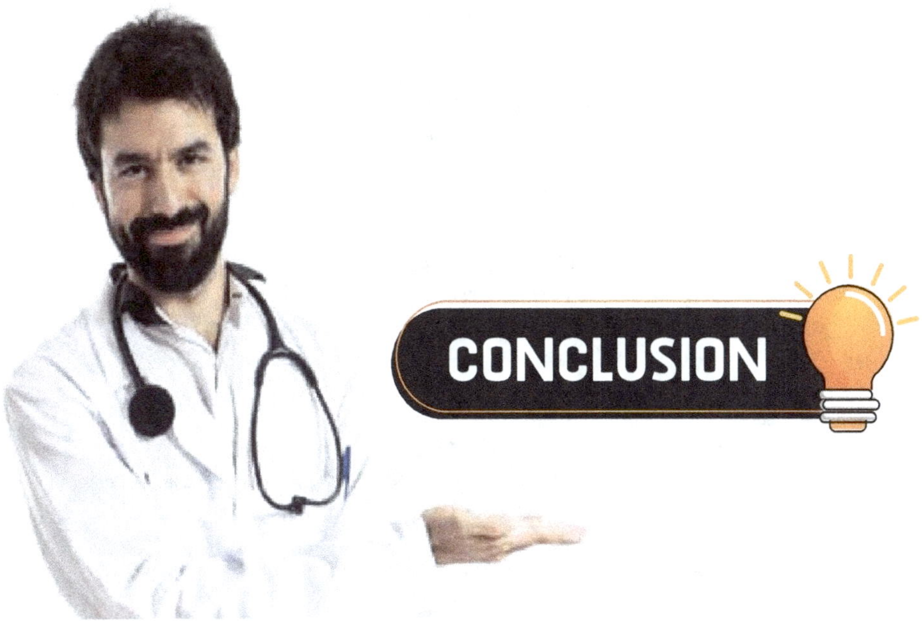

1- In brief, **cancer** is a complex disease that involves several dynamics.

These dynamics include oxidative damage, impaired DNA repair

mechanisms, DNA methylation and the killing of **cancer** cells by our

immune system.

2- Understanding these dynamics and working to oppose them can

help you defeat **cancer**.

Food can play a major role in your fight against **cancer**.

However, you need to always remember that the most important

component of your fight against cancer is to strongly believe that

you can defeat it as many already have!

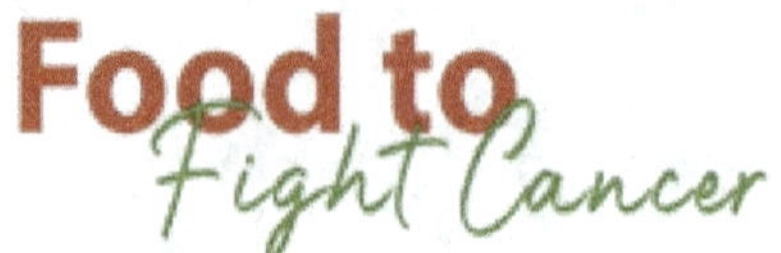

References

The Multi Dimensional Learning Model of Dr. Tarek M. Abdelhamid is available at
http://www.med-ed-online.org/t0000007.htm
http://www.ncbi.nlm.nih.gov/pmc/articles/PMC2515569/
http://www.cancer.gov/about-cancer/what-is-cancer#related-diseases
http://cancerres.aacrjournals.org/content/46/3/1015
http://www.cumc.columbia.edu/publications/in-vivo/Vol2_Iss10_may26_03/
http://www.ncbi.nlm.nih.gov/books/NBK9904/
http://www.cancer.org/acs/groups/cid/documents/webcontent/002550-pdf.pdf
http://study.com/academy/lesson/what-is-oxidation-definition-process-examples.html
http://www.ncbi.nlm.nih.gov/pmc/articles/PMC3249911/
http://www.ncbi.nlm.nih.gov/pmc/articles/PMC2684512/
http://www.ncbi.nlm.nih.gov/pmc/articles/PMC3249911/
http://www.ncbi.nlm.nih.gov/pubmed/20920744
http://www.sciencedirect.com/science/article/pii/S1357272599001399
http://www.sigmaaldrich.com/technical-documents/articles/biofiles/dna-damage-and-repair.html
http://www.ncbi.nlm.nih.gov/pmc/articles/PMC2657599/#R3
http://www.iflscience.com/watch-t-cells-hunt-down-and-kill-cancer-cells
http://www.ncbi.nlm.nih.gov/books/NBK21590/
http://www.ncbi.nlm.nih.gov/pmc/articles/PMC1993983/
http://www.medicalnewstoday.com/articles/283604.php
http://theoncologist.alphamedpress.org/content/6/3/298.full
http://www.ncbi.nlm.nih.gov/pmc/articles/PMC2802675/
http://www.ncbi.nlm.nih.gov/pmc/articles/PMC2224590/
http://www.cancer.gov/about-cancer/causes-prevention/risk/diet/cooked-meats-fact-sheet
http://www.nlm.nih.gov/medlineplus/ency/article/002096.htm
http://www.ncbi.nlm.nih.gov/books/NBK21551/
http://www.ncbi.nlm.nih.gov/pubmed/16550597
http://www.biomedcentral.com/content/pdf/1477-7819-12-164.pdf
http://www.pcrm.org/health/cancer-resources/diet-cancer/nutrition/how-fiber-helps-protect-against-cancer
http://jn.nutrition.org/content/134/12/3479S.full.pdf&member=&journal=nutrition&volume=134&issue_number=12&cover_date=December%201
http://health.clevelandclinic.org/2014/08/healthy-vitamin-d-levels-may-help-you-fight-cancer/
http://www.ncbi.nlm.nih.gov/pmc/articles/PMC2515569/
http://erc.endocrinology-journals.org/content/19/5/F27.full
http://researchnews.osu.edu/archive/ATF3.htm
http://www.todaysdietitian.com/newarchives/111609p38.shtml
http://www.oncologypractice.com/jso/journal/articles/0301037.pdf
http://www.ncbi.nlm.nih.gov/pubmed/18574467
http://www.ncbi.nlm.nih.gov/pmc/articles/PMC2840634/
https://books.google.com/books?id=5NbsAwAAQBAJ&pg=PA323&lpg=PA323&dq=anticancer+drugs+carcinogenesis+Robbins+pathologic+basis+of+disease&source=bl&ots=A49Hr1o0Dd&sig=lGK5f2w6JwrmS1wnAEKqehSeVBc&hl=en&sa=X&ved=0CB4Q6AEwAGoVChMljLz2svXaxgIVjn6SCh09hAxK#v=onepage&q=anticancer%20drugs%20carcinogenesis%20Robbins%20pathologic%20basis%20of%20disease&f=false

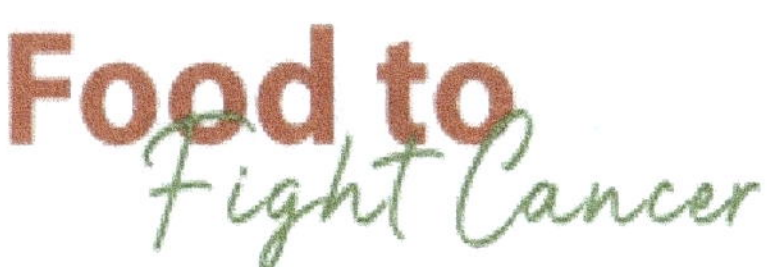

References

http://dictionary.reference.com/browse/detoxification
http://www.ncbi.nlm.nih.gov/pmc/articles/PMC2596047/
http://articles.mercola.com/sites/articles/archive/2010/04/10/can-you-use-food-to-increase-glutathione-instead-of-supplements.aspx
http://www.ncbi.nlm.nih.gov/pubmedhealth/PMH0032607/
http://www.ncbi.nlm.nih.gov/pubmed/11864778
http://www.huffingtonpost.com/dr-mark-hyman/glutathione-the-mother-of_b_530494.html
http://www.sciencedirect.com/science/article/pii/0006295281905219
http://articles.mercola.com/sites/articles/archive/2010/04/10/can-you-use-food-to-increase-glutathione-instead-of-supplements.aspx
http://www.inl.asia/resources-main-navigation-bar/the-liver-a-detoxification-part-2
http://www.inl.asia/resources-main-navigation-bar/the-liver-a-detoxification-part-2
http://www.inl.asia/resources-main-navigation-bar/the-liver-a-detoxification-part-2
http://www.inl.asia/resources-main-navigation-bar/the-liver-a-detoxification-part-2
http://www.ncbi.nlm.nih.gov/pmc/articles/PMC2515569/
http://umm.edu/health/medical/altmed/supplement/vitamin-c-ascorbic-acid
http://umm.edu/health/medical/altmed/supplement/vitamin-c-ascorbic-acid
http://www.ncbi.nlm.nih.gov/pmc/articles/PMC2040110/
http://www.lifeextension.com/magazine/2011/8/lipoic-acid-reverses-mitochondrial-decay/page-01
http://cms.herbalgram.org/herbalgram/issue62/article2696.html?ts=1436894171&signature=4d1f8d892 92c400e7326d9dea9d31ce6
http://www.ncbi.nlm.nih.gov/pmc/articles/PMC3736525/
http://www.ncbi.nlm.nih.gov/pubmed/16091010
http://www.ncbi.nlm.nih.gov/pmc/articles/PMC3757421/
http://www.lifeextension.com/Magazine/2008/2/Coenzyme-Q10-And-Cancer/Page-01
http://ajcn.nutrition.org/content/74/4/418.full
http://articles.mercola.com/sites/articles/archive/2013/10/28/resveratrol-cancer-prevention.aspx
http://www.ncbi.nlm.nih.gov/pubmed/1309685
http://www.ncbi.nlm.nih.gov/pubmed/1309685
http://www.ncbi.nlm.nih.gov/pmc/articles/PMC3543845/
http://www.ncbi.nlm.nih.gov/pmc/articles/PMC3032603/
http://www.ncbi.nlm.nih.gov/pubmed/25398691
http://www.ncbi.nlm.nih.gov/pmc/articles/PMC3081446/
http://jnci.oxfordjournals.org/content/95/2/98.long
http://www.wildwoodhealth.org/blog/cancer-prevention-strategies-dna-repair/
http://www.wildwoodhealth.org/blog/cancer-prevention-strategies-dna-repair/
http://www.news-medical.net/news/2006/02/14/15915.aspx
http://www.ncbi.nlm.nih.gov/pmc/articles/PMC3151020/
http://www.wildwoodhealth.org/blog/cancer-prevention-strategies-dna-repair/
http://jn.nutrition.org/content/132/8/2333S.short
http://www.news-medical.net/health/What-is-Folic-Acid.aspx
http://www.ncbi.nlm.nih.gov/pubmed/21152119
http://europepmc.org/abstract/med/10726985
http://www.ncbi.nlm.nih.gov/pmc/articles/PMC4369959/
http://www.pubfacts.com/detail/24051122/Ellagic-acid-induces-a-dose--and-time-dependent-depolarization-of-mitochondria-and-activation-of-cas
http://gww.ncbi.nlm.nih.gov/pubmed/24051122
http://jn.nutrition.org/content/136/11/2715.full
http://onlinelibrary.wiley.com/doi/10.1111/j.1600-0838.2005.00440.x/pdf
http://onlinelibrary.wiley.com/doi/10.1111/j.1440-1681.2005.04289.x/abstract
http://www.ncbi.nlm.nih.gov/pubmed/9927011

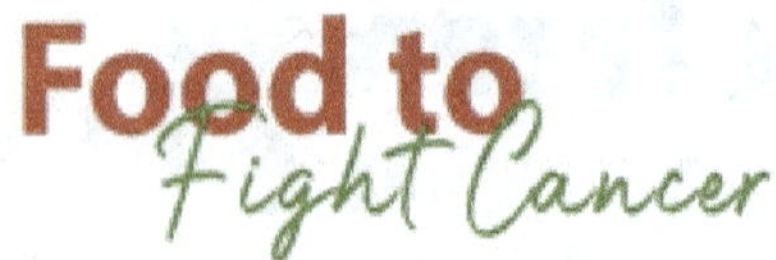

http://www.cancer.gov/about-cancer/treatment/types/surgery/hyperthermia-fact-sheet

http://jap.physiology.org/content/87/2/699

http://www.ncbi.nlm.nih.gov/pmc/articles/PMC1891166/

http://www.ncbi.nlm.nih.gov/books/NBK164700/

http://www.academicjournals.org/article/article1380188105_Rakashanda%20et%20al.pdf

http://www.ncbi.nlm.nih.gov/pmc/articles/PMC2862133/

http://thenational.net/lifestyle-health/sulforaphane-disease-fighting-compound-found-vegetables/4328/

http://thenational.net/lifestyle-health/sulforaphane-disease-fighting-compound-found-vegetables/4328/

http://www.aicr.org/foods-that-fight-cancer/foodsthatfightcancer_beans.html?referre
=https://www.google.com/

http://www.ncbi.nlm.nih.gov/pmc/articles/PMC4266039/

http://www.aicr.org/foods-that-fight-cancer/foodsthatfightcancer_beans.html?referrer
=https://www.google.com/

http://www.aicr.org/foods-that-fight-cancer/foodsthatfightcancer_beans.html?referrer
=https://www.google.com/

http://www.ncbi.nlm.nih.gov/pmc/articles/PMC3731019/

http://www.mdpi.com/1420-3049/19/2/2497

http://www.researchgate.net/publication/260378380_Effects_of_Honey_and_Its_Mechanisms_of_
Action_on_the_Development_and_Progression_of_Cancer

http://www.mdpi.com/1420-3049/19/2/2497

http://www.ncbi.nlm.nih.gov/pmc/articles/PMC3142888/

http://www.thelancet.com/journals/lanonc/article/PIIS1470-2045(00)00015-2/fulltext?version
=printerFriendly

http://www.tandfonline.com/doi/abs/10.1080/23723556.2015.1006077#.VaZQhvlViko

http://www.ncbi.nlm.nih.gov/pmc/articles/PMC3339609/

http://www.ncbi.nlm.nih.gov/pmc/articles/PMC3687424/

http://www.ncbi.nlm.nih.gov/pubmed/15584372

http://www.newsmax.com/Health/Cancer/Soybeans-Found-to-Have-Strong-Anti-Cancer-
Properties/2013/03/21/id/495790/

http://www.ncbi.nlm.nih.gov/pmc/articles/PMC3996758/

http://www.ncbi.nlm.nih.gov/pubmed/10726985

http://www.ncbi.nlm.nih.gov/pubmed/15137822

http://www.lookchem.com/Chempedia/Health-and-Chemical/18086.html

http://www.everydayhealth.com/depression-pictures/8-foods-that-fight-depression.aspx

https://www.ncbi.nlm.nih.gov/pmc/articles/PMC10080545/#:~:text=Chemical%20structure%20of%20
isolated%20constituents,and%20neuroprotective%20properties%5B22%5D.

https://pubmed.ncbi.nlm.nih.gov/29308747/

https://ar.iiarjournals.org/content/37/11/5995#:~:text=Their%20anticancer%20properties%20have%20
been,induction%20of%20cell%2Dcycle%20arrest.

https://www.ncbi.nlm.nih.gov/pmc/articles/PMC4163462/